T0290670

CONTROVERSIES
ON
COUNTERTRANSFERENCE

CONTROVERSIES
ON
COUNTERTRANSFERENCE

Edited by
Herbert S. Strean

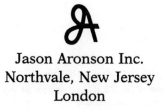

Jason Aronson Inc.
Northvale, New Jersey
London

This book was set in 11 pt. New Aster by Alabama Book Composition of Deatsville, AL, and printed and bound by Book-mart Press, Inc. of North Bergen, NJ.

Library of Congress Cataloging-in-Publication Data

Controversies on countertransference / edited by Herbert S. Strean.
    p. cm.
  Includes bibliographical references and index.
  ISBN 0-7657-0301-7
  1. Countertransference (Psychology) I. Strean, Herbert S.

  RC489.C68 C66 2000
  616.89'17-dc21

                             00-061063

Printed in the United States of America on acid-free paper. For information and catalog, write to Jason Aronson Inc., 230 Livingston Street, Northvale, NJ 07647-1726, or visit our website: www.aronson.com

To the discussants of this book:

Sally Barchilon
Jerrold Brandell
Gildo Consolini
James Hull
Michael Kasper
Harriet Klein
Jay Offen
Barbara Pizer
Angelo Smaldino
Martha Stark
Stanley Teitelbaum
Stephen Weiss

good friends and valued colleagues who gave so generously
and made this book become a reality.

Contents

Preface

As I reflect on my half century's experience as a psychotherapist, I see that very few subjects have stimulated, challenged, and affected me more than countertransference. Whether it was fantasies, reactions, or behaviors toward one of my own patients or that of my colleagues or students, confronting countertransference issues, understanding them, and mastering them has been a life-long task and will continue to be so.

Like those trained in the early 1950s, I was taught to believe that "countertransference" was a dirty word, and to reveal any sign of it to anyone was like acknowledging that one had a serious disease. Several incidents come to mind. It was 1953 and I was an army officer during the Korean War, functioning as a clinician and supervisor in a mental hygiene clinic at Fort Dix, New Jersey. While interviewing a paranoid soldier who was in the midst of a psychotic break, I found myself rapidly moving one of my feet back and forth. As I was taking note of my symptomatic act, my patient simultaneously commented, "You want to kick me out, don't you?" Embarrassed, ashamed, and guilty, I kept quiet, and my patient did a wonderful job of berating me! I later shared the experience with my supervisor, who responded by saying,

"You have to monitor your aggression better than you do!" I felt like saying to him, "And so do you!" but I didn't.

A few years later, while in training to become a child analyst, I put my arm around a 4-year-old boy who was crying because his mother had been abruptly taken to the hospital. With my arm still around him I said, "Tony, I feel very sorry for you and I'll do my best to be near you until Mommy comes home." When I reported my intervention to an analytic seminar, I was castigated by everyone, particularly the leader, for "acting out" my "overidentification" and "not relating to his intrapsychic conflict."

Still later, when I told my control analyst that a patient in my private practice was rushed to a hospital for an emergency appendectomy and that I telephoned there, he suggested that I "contaminated the transference, compounded the patient's resistance, and relinquished the anonymous neutral abstinent role."

All of these incidents made me question my therapeutic competence and for a long time caused me to idealize the role of the non-feeling clinician who mirrors and interprets his or her patient's conflicts.

Yet, I never felt comfortable trying to deny and repress my countertransference reactions. As I continued to experience a wide range of feelings toward my patients, such as love, hatred, ambivalence, sexual and aggressive fantasies, and more, it slowly began to dawn on me that I was having unique reactions to unique patients. Although I studied my idiosyncratic responses to my patients in my personal analysis, in supervision, and on my own, I began to realize that maybe what my patients induced in me told me not only something about myself, but something about them, too. For example, maybe the woman who induced strong erotic fantasies in me wanted me to feel sexually excited because it did something for her. Maybe the gentleman with whom I found myself competing wanted to engage me in some rivalry.

As I continued to study my countertransference reactions and could separate more and more what the patient induced in me from my own history and dynamics (and what I tended to induce in others), I began to frame many of my interventions by my countertransference responses with very satisfying therapeutic results.

I remember coming to the conclusion in the 1970s that every therapeutic intervention emanates from the therapist's countertransference position. And I began to observe in my colleagues, students, and supervisees what I noticed in myself: the more we practitioners confront, acknowledge, and analyze countertransference reactions, the more we are able to conduct sensitive, empathetic therapy that helps the patient grow in significant ways.

As I read the literature from object relations, self psychology, and intersubjective theorists, I also concluded that to understand what happens in psychotherapy, we have to utilize a two-person psychology. By a two-person psychology I mean that in the therapeutic situation there are always two vulnerable individuals present who are constantly affecting the therapeutic outcome through their interaction. By 1980, I deemed the notion of the wise, together therapist ministering to the weak disorganized patient unrealistic. I became enamored with Harry Stack Sullivan's perspective that therapist and patient "are more human than otherwise."

With the firm conviction that therapist and patient are equals who are trying their best to have a meaningful dialogue, I began to share some of my countertransference reactions with my patients. At first I did this when I found that conventional procedures (for example, interpretation, clarification, and confrontation) were not achieving very good therapeutic results. To my delight, I found and still find that when resistances and transference issues are not being resolved, disclosure of selected countertransference responses tends to clarify the transference, resolve resistances, and strengthen the therapeutic alliance. Today I frequently share

countertransference responses when I am asked for them
and/or when I believe they will enhance the therapy.

The chapters in this book reflect my struggles and
triumphs in dealing with countertransference issues. These
chapters were originally articles I wrote that were published
in various clinical journals and are reports of ongoing discoveries and shifts in my therapeutic stance. Inasmuch as all of
the chapters in this book, when originally published, stimulated much controversy, I thought it would be helpful not only
to republish most of the countertransference articles I have
written, but to try to replicate the debates and discussions
that I had with colleagues.

Because I am convinced that honest debate and discussion, without vitriolic and combative language, can enhance
the work of mental health professionals, I have asked colleagues who have taken positions on countertransference
issues—often different from my own—to write responses to
the six papers I have chosen to replicate in this book.

My selection of discussants was far from arbitrary. All of
them have had twenty or more years of experience practicing
and teaching psychotherapy. All of them have been part of the
changing landscape in psychotherapy and have struggled to
take clearly articulated positions on countertransference.
When the chapter under discussion is on theoretical predilections, the discussants are very much interested in theoretical
issues. If the topic is supervision, training, or therapeutic
technique, the discussants have considerable expertise in
these areas.

I am extremely grateful to the twelve colleagues who
have made the publication of this book possible. I also want to
thank the many patients, supervisees, and students who
helped me formulate and reformulate the ideas presented in
this book.

My wife, Marcia, has consistently and compassionately
edited, typed, and reviewed all of my written work for well

over four decades and I want to express my abiding gratitude and love to her. Finally, to Dr. Jason Aronson and all of my friends at Jason Aronson, Inc., Norma Pomerantz and Judy Cohen, it's a pleasure working with you.

Herbert S. Strean
January 2001

About the Discussants

Sally Barchilon, M.S.W., is Director of the Hudson Valley Division of the New York Center for Psychoanalytic Training, where she is also a training analyst, supervisor, and faculty member. She is on the faculty of Hunter School of Social Work, and is a consultant and seminar leader at several treatment centers and social agencies.

Jerrold R. Brandell, Ph.D., is Professor of Social Work, Wayne State University, Detroit, Michigan, where he chairs the Graduate Concentration in Mental Health and teaches courses on child and adult psychopathology and clinical treatment. An advanced candidate in psychoanalysis, he has published four books, including *Of Mice and Metaphors: Therapeutic Storytelling with Children,* and *Countertransference in Psychotherapy with Children and Adolescents,* and is a founding editor of the clinical quarterly *Psychoanalytic Social Work.* Dr. Brandell is currently Chair of the Study Group of the National Membership Committee on Psychoanalysis. He resides in Ann Arbor, Michigan, where he maintains a part-time private practice and is actively involved in clinical supervision and consultation.

Gildo Consolini, M.S.W., practices psychotherapy, psychoanalysis, and marriage counseling privately in New York City.

He is a training analyst at the New York Center for Psycho-analytic Training, lecturer at the Shirley M. Ehrenkranz School of Social Work of New York University, and has published papers in the *Clinical Social Work Journal* and the *Journal of Analytic Social Work*.

James W. Hull, Ph.D., is a psychoanalyst in private practice. He is on the faculty of Cornell Medical College and is a training analyst and faculty member at the New York Center for Psychoanalytic Training. Dr. Hull has written several articles and book chapters on psychoanalysis and psycho-therapy.

Michael Kasper, M.S.W., is on the faculty and is a training analyst at the New York Center for Psychoanalytic Training. He is also on the faculty of the Post-Masters program in clinical social work at Hunter College. Mr. Kasper practices psychotherapy and psychoanalysis in New York City and Rockland County.

Harriet Klein, M.S.W., is an analyst in private practice in New York City. She is a training analyst and supervisor at the New York Center for Psychoanalytic Training. She has served as a member of the NYCPT Board of Directors and Training Committee and was previously a supervisor for the Veterans Administration Hospital in New York City.

Jay Rae Offen, M.S.W., is a practicing psychoanalyst in New York City and Nyack, NY. She is a training analyst at the New York Center for Psychoanalytic Training, co-founder of the Hudson Valley Division of NYCPT, and a faculty member there. Her writing has appeared in several psychoanalytic journals.

Barbara Pizer, Ed.D., ABPP, is faculty and supervising analyst at the Massachusetts Institute for Psychoanalysis, faculty, The Psychoanalytic Institute of Northern California, member, of the New York Freudian Society and the International Psychoanalytic Association, clinical instructor in Psychology at Harvard Medical School, secretary of the Academy of Psychoanalysis, and author of numerous articles and chapters on the analyst's use of self, the technique of self-disclosure, and the body in psychoanalysis.

Angelo Smaldino, Ph.D., JD, is a training and control analyst at the National Psychological Association of Psychoanalysis and the New York Center for Psychoanalytic Training. He is past Dean of Training at NYCPT and author of papers on addiction and related subjects. Editor of the book *Psychoanalytic Approaches to Addiction*, he is in private practice in New York City and Port Washington, Long Island.

Martha Stark, M.D., is a training and supervising analyst at the Boston Psychoanalytic Institute. She has a teaching appointment at the Massachusetts Mental Health Center and is a clinical instructor in psychiatry at Harvard Medical School. Among her many publications are *Working with Resistance, A Primer on Working with Resistance*, and *Modes of Therapeutic Action*.

Stanley H. Teitelbaum, Ph.D., is the author of the recently published *Illusion and Disillusionment: Core Issues in Psychotherapy*. Dr. Teitelbaum is Director of the Training Program in Supervision of the Psychoanalytic Process at the Postgraduate Center for Mental Health where he also serves as a training analyst, senior supervisor, and faculty member. He is Dean of Training at the Contemporary Center for Advanced Psychoanalytic Studies. Widely published in professional journals, Dr. Teitelbaum is best known for his writings in the field of psychoanalytic supervision.

Stephen G. Weiss, Ph.D., is Associate Professor and Director of the Program in Early Childhood and Elementary Education at New York University. In the past, he has been Director of the Program Preparing Teachers of Emotionally Disturbed Children and Director of the Commission on Special Education at New York University. Dr. Weiss is an associate member at the New York Center for Psychoanalytic Training where he holds a certificate in psychoanalytic psychotherapy. He is in private practice with children, adolescents, and adults in New York City.

1

Countertransference:
An Introduction

WHAT IS COUNTERTRANSFERENCE?

The controversial nature of countertransference is best revealed when we confront its definitions. The first clinician to offer a definition of the term was Sigmund Freud. In his paper, "The Future Prospects of Psycho-Analytic Therapy" (1910), Freud wrote:

> We have become aware of the "counter-transference" which arises in [the patient's influence on his therapist] as a result of the patient's influence on his unconscious feelings and we are almost inclined to insist that he shall recognize this counter-transference in himself and overcome it. We have noticed that no psychoanalyst goes further than his own complexes and resistances permit, and we consequently require that he shall begin his activity with a self-analysis

and continually carry it deeper while he is making his own observations on his patients. [pp. 144–145]

Freud's definition of countertransference has served as an ideal for many psychotherapists, regardless of their theoretical predilections or clinical biases. In *Psychoanalytic Terms and Concepts*, published eighty years after Freud presented his definition of countertransference, Moore and Fine (1990) defined countertransference as

a situation in which an analyst's feelings and attitudes toward a patient are derived from earlier situations in the analyst's life that have been displaced onto the patient. Countertransference therefore reflects the analyst's own unconscious reaction to the patient, though some aspects may be conscious. [p. 47]

It would appear that Moore and Fine's definition of countertransference very much reflects Freud's advice to therapists, which is to model themselves after the surgeon "who puts aside all of his feelings, even his human sympathy, and concentrates his mental forces on the single aim of performing the operation as skillfully as possible" (1912b, p. 105). The justification for requiring this emotional detachment in the therapist is that it creates the most advantageous conditions for both parties. It is considered to be a desirable protection for the practitioner's own emotional life and it ensures the patient available help.

In 1912 Freud added the following remarks to his definition of countertransference:

To put into a formula: [the therapist] must turn his own unconscious like a receptive organ toward the transmitting unconscious of the patient. He must adjust himself to the patient as a telephone receiver is adjusted to the transmitting microphone. Just as the receiver converts back into soundwave the electric oscillations . . . so the doctor's unconscious is able, from the derivatives of the unconscious which are communicated to him, to reconstruct the unconscious, which has determined the patient's free associations. [1912a, pp. 111–112]

As we reflect on Freud's 1910 and 1912 definitions of countertransference, these quotations demonstrate a fundamental contradiction. First Freud suggests that the clinician be like "a surgeon," "a mirror," "an instrument," but then suggests that the clinician react with his own unconscious to the patient. Freud concomitantly excludes and includes the practitioner's subjective and emotional life.

While the Moore and Fine (1990) definition of countertransference mirrors Freud's of 1910, many contemporary clinicians agree with the way Freud, in 1912, regarded the unconscious of the therapist as something that always influences the patient's unconscious communications.

Slakter (1987) pointed out that countertransference, rather than an obstacle to be overcome, is to be regarded as "all those reactions (of the therapist) to the patient that may help or hinder treatment" (p. v). Abend (1989) suggested that current clinicians tend to view countertransference as including "all of the emotional reactions [of the therapist] at work" (p. 374) and Epstein and Feiner (1979) concluded:

Countertransference is now seen as a normal, natural interpersonal event, rather than as an idiosyncratic pathological phenomenon. This has facilitated the shift from viewing countertransference reactions solely as a hindrance, to viewing them for their potential value in understanding the patient and the therapeutic relationship, and in formulating inter-

ventions which deepen and intensify the psychotherapeutic process. [p. 19]

THE THERAPIST'S STRUGGLE (1910–2001)

The varied definitions of countertransference reflect rather
clearly, I believe, the struggle every practicing clinician has,
starting with Freud and continuing into the present. It will
always be a struggle for practitioners to cope with their
subjective reactions in therapy on one hand and to use them
constructively to facilitate treatment on the other.

The difficulty in coping with countertransference is best
exemplified by Freud himself. Although his idealized image of
the clinician was that of the dispassionate surgeon who
performs his work unemotionally, diligently, and objectively,
Freud did not usually behave this way with his patients. Freud
lent money to patients, fed some, hugged others, gave advice
to many, and even took some patients with him on vacation
(Jones 1953, Strean 1993). Although his adherents constantly
parroted Freud's notion of the dispassionate surgeon who
must relinquish his subjectivity, like the master, they did not
practice what they preached. Otto Rank turned his analysand,
Anais Nin, into his mistress. Ernest Jones, Freud's biographer,
spent a good part of his career fending off accusations that he
sexually molested young patients and had sexual intercourse
with older ones. Carl Jung had prolonged affairs with several
of his patients, including one who became a psychoanalyst.
And Sandor Ferenczi believed that his patients needed physical comfort; therefore, he openly fondled their breasts and
frequently hugged them (Grosskurth 1991).

When Freud's colleague, Dr. Josef Breuer, noted that his
patient, Anna O., lusted after him and wanted him to father
her fantasied baby, he stopped her treatment and abruptly
went off on a second honeymoon with his wife and had a baby
with her (Breuer and Freud 1936). When Freud observed

what happened to his colleague, he probably avoided confronting his own countertransference responses and hence did not write very much on the subject. It is rather fascinating that in contrast to his meticulous discussions of transference, Freud wrote next to nothing on countertransference. In the twenty-four volumes of the *Standard Edition*, there are only four references to countertransference. Like Freud, many contemporary clinicians avoid dialogues on countertransference issues and instead discuss, at great length and almost exclusively, the transference reactions, resistance, and dynamics of their patients.

I would guess that all therapists experience Freud's dilemma at some time in their careers. Inasmuch as the psychotherapeutic encounter is an intense, intimate one for both parties, it is very tempting to act out erotic and aggressive impulses, either directly or indirectly. When the temptation is great and the anxiety is high, an understandable defense is for the therapist to say to himself or herself: "My countertransference wishes don't exist. I feel nothing but objective." On the other hand, like many of Freud's followers who felt obliged to obey the master's prescriptions and be a dispassionate surgeon—something they found too difficult at times and rebelled against—many contemporary clinicians feel impelled to act upon their countertransference wishes with their patients (Strean 1993). It has been a difficult task for most of us to be aware of and monitor our countertransference responses and concomitantly utilize them in the treatment situation to the patient's advantage. This is particularly difficult because as Renik (1993a) has clearly demonstrated, "awareness of countertransference is always retrospective, preceded by countertransference enactment" (p. 556). It is only after the countertransference enactment that the clinician may become aware of the nature of his personal involvement.

Because countertransference reactions are always being aroused and inasmuch as we are always tempted to act upon them without knowing their unconscious significance, it is difficult to find the middle ground and be a feeling, reacting, subjective therapist who is at the same time empathetic and always working on the patient's behalf.

MOVES TOWARD THE MIDDLE GROUND

One of the first to broaden the operational definition of countertransference was Ferenczi (1919). As recorded in his diary of 1932 and published in 1988, Ferenczi averred: "One could almost say that the more weaknesses an analyst has, which lead to great or lesser mistakes and errors but which are then uncovered and treated in the course of mutual analysis, the more likely the analysis is to rest on profound and realistic foundations" (p. 15).

Ferenczi was one of the first clinicians to point out emphatically that the practitioner was first and foremost a human being and that his reactions are inevitably part of the therapeutic process. Soon after Ferenczi presented some of his ideas on countertransference, Stern (1924) took the position that the therapeutic process is enhanced when the clinician can identify with the patient's transference. When the therapist is able to do so, his own countertransference responses will not be as much of an interference. Helene Deutsch (1926) suggested that the clinician should identify emotionally with the patient's infantile ego and in doing this can, as Stern suggested, not be as influenced by idiosyncratic subjective countertransference reactions. In 1927, Glover pointed out that the practitioner's countertransference responses are always influenced by the patient's transference reactions and vice versa. Strachey (1934) referred to this process or interaction as "mutuality" in which therapist and patient are always influencing each other.

Low (1935) suggested that the clinician's contact with his own emotions leads to the insights that help the patient feel understood and able to make efforts to change. Balint and Balint (1939) discussed the impact the clinician's personality and history have on the patient's transference reactions. How therapists dress, furnish their offices, begin and end sessions, seize on certain material, such as dreams, all influence the patient's transference reactions, which in turn reinforce or weaken certain countertransference responses.

The mutual effect that patient and therapist have on each other has been referred to as the intersubjective perspective (Natterson 1991, Stolorow 1984, Stolorow and Atwood 1979, 1984). One of the first intersubjective innovators was Franz Alexander (Alexander and French 1946), who developed the concept of the *corrective emotional experience*. In this experience cure is understood to arise from a specific role that the therapist selects to enact with the patient, different from what the patient's unhappy life experience has been with previous role partners. This corrective role is developed by first studying very carefully the spontaneous interaction between patient and therapist.

UTILIZING THE COUNTERTRANSFERENCE WITH THE PATIENT

By the 1950s, therapists were freeing themselves of the view that countertransference was something bad and not to be discussed with colleagues or revealed to patients. Paula Heimann (1950) not only extended the notion of countertransference to include all of the feelings that the therapist experiences, no longer restricting it to the pathological, as Freud did, but she considered the practitioner's emotional response to the patient as one of the most important tools for therapeutic work. Stated Heimann: "The analyst's countertransference is an instrument of research into the patient's unconscious" (p. 81).

Margaret Little (1951) placed the therapist's countertransference at the center of therapeutic work, particularly with severely disturbed patients. She pointed out that severely disturbed patients are often successfully treated by beginning therapists who are not afraid to allow their unconscious impulses to be explored. I was able to replicate this finding in the 1970s when I learned that the best therapists for in-patient schizophrenics are first-year social work students. Unencumbered by the cynicism that many experienced clinicians demonstrate, they relate to these disturbed patients in a warm, spontaneous, humane manner and often achieve much better results than their more experienced counterparts (Strean 1982).

It was Frieda Fromm-Reichmann (1950), like Little, who suggested that to be helpful and achieve therapeutic results with very disturbed patients, the therapist must share some of her spontaneous emotions. D.W. Winnicott (1949) supported Little's and Fromm-Reichmann's sentiment. He suggested that if a clinician is to do good therapeutic work with psychotic or anitisocial patients, "he must be able to be so thoroughly aware of the countertransference that he can sort out and study his objective reactions to the patient. These will include hate" (p. 70).

Winnicott was one of the first clinicians to feel it was appropriate to share his hateful feelings with the patient at specific times. He believed that by doing so the patient could eventually get in touch with his own hatred and its genetic roots. If practitioners did not feel their hatred in the countertransference (and other emotional reactions such as envy, love, ambivalence, and so forth) in the countertransference they would be showing the patient their "false selves" and thus would encourage the patient to be less authentic.

Heinrich Racker (1968) demonstrated how under certain conditions therapists can find themselves in the psychological position of the child next to the patient, who is experienced as a mother or a father. Racker referred to this phenomenon as *the countertransference neurosis* and suggested that it is as inevitable in the clinician as the transference neurosis is in the patient. According to Racker, countertransference is the most reliable guide to knowing what the therapist should respond to in the patient's communications or behavior at any given moment.

From 1910 to 1950, particularly from the 1940s on, many clinicians began to acknowledge the inevitability of counter-transference, use it in understanding patients, plan therapeu-tic interventions around it, and at times share it with the patient. However, many other practitioners continued to subscribe to Freud's 1910 definition of countertransference. One of the leading spokespersons who continued to maintain that countertransference was always pathological and always interfered with therapeutic progress was Annie Reich (1951, 1966). She sharply rejected the notion that countertransfer-ence could in any way be utilized as a therapeutic tool, either for understanding or for communicating with the patient. She averred that to use the clinician's countertransference experi-ences to understand the patient was really a poor substitute for empathy (1951). In all of her papers she made a strong plea for clinicians to do everything they could to remain uninvolved.

DEFINITIONS OF COUNTERTRANSFERENCE EXPAND

In his review of the literature on countertransference, Otto Kernberg (1965) used the term *classicist* to refer to Freud's original definition of countertransference, and the term *totalist* to refer to the broader views we have been considering in this chapter.

A classicist point of view, according to Kernberg, em-ploys the term countertransference to refer to the clinician's unresolved conflicts that are aroused by the patient's trans-ference and that can hinder the therapy. For some classical psychoanalysts, noting countertransference as a problem to be resolved through further personal analysis is the limit of its function (Fliess 1953) and sharing a countertransference reaction with a patient is considered a technical error (Reich 1960).

Totalist therapists, Kernberg suggests, have a broader definition in mind. To them, countertransference includes all the emotional responses the therapist has during the therapy. Totalists tend to view the source of countertransference phenomena as the interaction between patient and therapist, therefore involving both. Although many countertransference responses may be a function of unconscious factors, conscious experience is also taken into account and used as a source of information about the patient and the therapist. Hence, totalists are interested in a more comprehensive exploration of the clinician's feelings, reactions, and identifications in an attempt to obtain information about the patient and the therapeutic interaction.

According to Mendelsohn and colleagues (1992), totalists seem to be suggesting that all reactions are countertransferential. They add:

> [C]lassicist analysts sometimes sound like totalists while totalist analysts can sound like their classicist counterparts. Thus, Greenson (1967), a classical analyst, has proposed the following: "In order to listen effectively one must also pay attention to one's own emotional responses since these responses often lead to important clues." On the other hand, a noted totalist, Heimann (1950), states the following: "the approach to the countertransference is not without danger," while another totalist, Issacharoff (1976), states: "the indiscriminate use of countertransference material become reminiscent of the dangers of wild analysis." [p. 366]

In 1970 Sandler and colleagues summarized the various meanings of countertransference that were predominant in the literature at that time: (1) the resistances of the therapist resulting from the activation of unresolved conflicts by the patient's material, (2) the therapist's transference, (3) the therapist's characteristics of personality reflected in his work, which may or may not cause difficulties in the treatment process, (4) the totality of the therapist's unconscious attitudes toward his patients, (5) the therapist's "blind spots," (6) the therapist's conscious and unconscious reaction to the patient's transference, and (7) the "normal" or appropriate emotional response of the therapist to his patient.

Epstein and Feiner (1979) identify four working orientations to countertransference used by different therapists:

1. Countertransference is attended to when "difficulties arise," when the therapist experiences emotional disturbances, or disturbances of attention or concentration. Such interferences are then subjected to self-analysis.
2. Interferences in the analyst's efforts caused by disturbances in the analyst's emotional state are studied primarily in order to gain an understanding of the patient's contribution.
3. The totality of the countertransference is used as essential data for understanding the patient in the here and now. Accordingly, the countertransference is frequently considered when formulating interventions and strategies. Interventions may be restricted to interpretations; countertransference fantasies may be directly communicated to the patient; or induced countertransference feelings may be communicated "as needed" by the patient. This orientation usually includes the view that the therapist's internal silent processing of countertransferential disturbances is essential to the further integration of the patient. This

is seen as especially important with the more disturbed patient.

4. Countertransference inevitably infiltrates the patient's unconscious processes. Such infiltrations must be constantly monitored by studying the patient's associations and responses, and subsequently interpreted. [pp. 12–13]

THERAPIST AND PATIENT BECOME EQUALS

In 1974 Ralph Greenson pointed out that the therapeutic relationship could not be viewed as merely consisting of transferences of the patient toward the clinician. He stressed that there is a genuine, realistic, non-fantasy relationship between therapist and patient, and this relationship plays an essential role in resolving the transference neurosis. Greenson was convinced that interpretation without a warm, human interaction will not resolve emotional and interpersonal problems. The relationship that Greenson has described occurs on many occasions when the therapist is not neutral or objective, but instead is a real partner in a joint venture.

In 1977, Feiner referred to the ultimate extension of Freud's ideas on self-analysis, and stated that the key to the analysis of the patient resides in the analysis of the analyst. In this process, Feiner suggests, the clinician should partially dispense with the traditional requirement of differentiating between what is usable and what is not. In effect, the usable, or normal, elements in the practitioner's character structure are interwoven with the unusable or neurotic elements.

Similar to Greenson's (1967) notion of "the real relationship," Issacharoff and Hunt (1978) introduced the term *beyond countertransference* to refer to the shared experience that constitutes the therapeutic relationship. This term aims to help equalize the relationship between practitioner and patient.

Harold Searles (1975) suggested that there is an element of reality in all of the patient's distorted transference perceptions of the therapist. He further suggested that once the patient begins to understand some of the therapist's unconscious conflicts, she will often try to act as the therapist's therapist and help him become better attuned to the patient's struggles.

In 1959, while a student in psychoanalytic training and aware that many of my patients knew what they needed from the therapeutic relationship with me, I wrote a paper (1970) entitled "The Use of the Patient as Consultant." Here I presented three cases of patients who prescribed the kind of therapeutic relationship they needed from me and that I later provided. Their prescriptions and my adhering to them led to a resolution of several of their conflicts. In many ways, my efforts validate Searles's postulates. He was the first to see how the therapist's failure to recognize the countertransference could, like a mother's poor relationship to her child, stunt the patient's development into an autonomous individual.

Karl Menninger (1973) pointed out that countertransference is dangerous only when it is overlooked by the practitioner. He distinguished between countertransference that arose in the clinician's work over and over again and that which took place only with a specific patient. He believed that when countertransference is recognized by the therapist and not resisted, the patient's transference is almost always better understood by both members of the therapeutic dyad. When countertransference is unrecognized, the therapist could behave in ways that might undermine the treatment.

Peter Giovacchini (1979), who has specialized in treating very disturbed individuals, points out that psychotic patients are particularly adept in stimulating disruptive impulses in the therapist. Because these patients activate so much anxiety in clinicians, some therapists declare that they are untreatable, in order to protect themselves against feeling the discomfort. Giovacchini believes that only by acknowledging countertransference feelings and sharing them with the disturbed patient can the patient be helped.

Charles Brenner (1985) pointed out that countertransference is really the transference of the therapist in the treatment situation and therefore there is no need for a separate term. This same sentiment was voiced by McLaughlin (1981). Brenner has posited that countertransference is what makes a therapist's professional activity possible. Were it not for the fact that being a clinician offers each of us the particular combination of drive gratification, defense, and superego functioning that is characteristic for our particular compromise formations, none of us would be therapists. Martin Silverman (1985) stresses that the therapist is no less human than the patient and therefore is full of anxieties, vulnerabilities, and idiosyncrasies. He suggests that unless clinicians can genuinely acknowledge their pathological parts, they will limit or destroy their efforts to help patients overcome the neurotic problems that are preventing them from realizing their potential in life.

Sandler (1976), like many of his contemporaries, stressed the theme of equality between practitioner and patient. He demonstrated that both patient and therapist are unconsciously striving to induce the other to enact different roles. How much both parties are willing to complement each other in their interaction will, in many ways, determine the therapeutic outcome. The notion of role induction and role reciprocity was originally introduced by Marie Coleman Nelson and colleagues in 1968. In addition to what Sandler prescribed, Nelson suggested that the therapist enact specific roles to resolve certain transference–countertransference difficulties.

Starting in the 1960s and continuing into the present, many therapists have accentuated the significance of countertransference being as inevitable as transference. This sentiment is well stated by Searles (1987):

I can believe that the time will come, in our work with neurotic patients, when, just as we now use as a criterion of analyzability the patient's capability for developing a transference neurosis, we may use as an additional criterion of earlier predictive significance in our work with the patient, his capability in fostering a countertransference neurosis, so to speak, in the analyst. [p. 146]

DISCLOSING THE COUNTERTRANSFERENCE TO THE PATIENT

During the last few years clinicians have not only viewed countertransference as ever-present in the therapeutic situation, to be used as an indicator of the patient's dynamics, particularly his transference, but as something to be shared with the patient to clarify the transference, resolve resistances, and strengthen the therapeutic alliance. One of the first writers to consider disclosing countertransference responses was Theodore Jacobs. Jacobs pointed out that whether overt or disguised, dramatic or barely perceptible, the therapist's transference may exert a significant influence not only on his observations and understanding but on the particular form and manner in which the patient's transferences emerge. States Jacobs (1986):

The way in which we listen, our silences and neutrality; the emphasis we place on transference phenomena and interpretation of the transference; our ideas concerning working through, termination and what constitutes a "correct" interpretation; these and many other facets of our daily clinical work may, and not infrequently do, contain within them concealed countertransference elements. [p. 166]

In a more recent paper, Jacobs (1999) discusses different types of self-disclosure. Alluded to above are those disclosures that occur outside of the clinician's awareness through slips, errors, and by other nonverbal means. Then there are those kinds of self-disclosure that involve deliberate acts on the part of the clinician: sharing with patients certain subjective experiences and answering particular types of questions. Jacobs has demonstrated that the therapeutic work frequently can be enhanced rather than compromised when the therapist answers questions and shares certain feelings or fantasies, particularly as they are experienced in the therapeutic interaction. As Jacobs (1999) points out:

> In certain individuals—for instance, those who have had long experiences with secretive, non-responsive parents or whose self-esteem is particularly fragile— the traditional analytic attitude with regard to self-disclosure may be experienced as hostile and may have an inhibiting effect rather than being liberating. Instead of functioning to open up communications and to free up the mind, it can shut it down. [p. 164]

Jacobs repeats the point that whether we disclose countertransference responses and when depends on the patient and the material at hand. Patients who have not experienced affective interactions with parents and others often profit very much from a therapist who discloses some of her affects as they emerge in the therapy.

Another prominent contributor to the literature on the therapist's self-disclosure is Renik (1993a,b, 1995). Like Jacobs, he proposes that all of the therapist's activity emanates from his current countertransference position, and the subjectivity of the clinician is always present. Furthermore, Renik demonstrates that the therapist's subjectivity can only be discovered in hindsight. He makes an excellent case in demonstrating that there is no such thing as the neutral, abstinent anonymous therapist. Renik (1999) champions a policy of consistent willingness on the clinician's part to make his own views explicitly available to the patient. By playing one's cards face up, Renik departs from Jacobs's position and the position of most clinicians who selectively make self-disclosures of their countertransference reactions. Renik is able to demonstrate clearly that consistent authenticity helps create a candid dialogue, thus facilitating maximally effective collaboration between therapist and patient. He says: "the benefit of an analyst's willingness to self-disclose is that it establishes the analyst's fallible view of his or her own participation in the analysis as an appropriate subject for collaborative investigation—something analyst and patient can and should talk about explicitly together" (p. 529).

The clinician who has written the most on self-disclosure is Karen Maroda. Through many case examples (Maroda 1994) she shows how the therapist's neutrality can be used in practice as a place for the therapist to hide from the patient. She clearly explicates how one can enter into the role assigned by the patient (Sandler 1976), and then, through reflective disclosure, help the patient to find an alternative to the dysfunctional patterns of the past. Like Jacobs and Renik, Maroda is convinced that the psychotherapeutic process consists of two participants in mutual interaction and that both parties bring to the relationship their own wishes, fantasies, defenses, hopes, and fears. Maroda (1994, 1999) demonstrates how her immediate emotional reaction to the patient is the most important disclosure to reveal and that personal information about her own life is often unnecessary. Using her patients as consultants, Maroda times her self-disclosures and their nature by listening carefully to what her patients show her they need and when they need it.

Maroda also discusses the misuse of self-disclosure, when it is used to further the therapist's personal or professional agenda. This includes seductive disclosures of love or sexual attraction by the therapist, when the patient was *not* seeking this information; unsolicited expressions of the clinician's feelings of inadequacy, particularly when paired with idealizing comments about the patient; attempting to express intense feelings when the therapist is feeling out of control; and giving in and masochistically submitting to a sadistic patient who is demanding love or some other indulgence. Maroda gives clinical examples of her own misuse of self-disclosure, such as when she expressed love to a patient who did not solicit it and in another case when she expressed admiration to a patient who did not request it. Maroda demonstrates in all of her work how patients respond to and experience the therapist's self-disclosure. Maroda's work is a contribution that emanates from a relatively new perspective called *relational theory*. Stimulated by the work of Stephen Mitchell (1988) and Lewis Aron (1996), relational theory is based on the shift from the classical psychoanalytic notion that it is the patient's mind that is being studied to the relational idea that the mind is social, interactional, and interpersonal. This distinction between the classical and relational views is often what is implied when we discuss the shift from a one-person to a two-person psychology.

What the relational theorists emphasize is their understanding that "transference is not simply a distortion that emerges or unfolds from within the patient, independent of the actual behavior and personality of the analyst. Rather, the analyst is viewed as a participant in the analysis whose behavior has an interpersonal impact on the cocreation or construction of the transference" (Aron 1996, pp. 11–12).

Giovacchini (1993) like Maroda, believes that disclosure of the countertransference is most helpful to the therapeutic process when the patient is overtly or covertly trying to defeat the therapist. Giovacchini shows that the patient can often acknowledge her transference projections only if the therapist can first admit to his countertransference responses.

The notion of the countertransference as something bad

and to be overcome, although still somewhat in vogue, has been dramatically modified in the last several decades. As clinicians recognize the universality and ever-presence of countertransference and are freer to share it with their patients (Renik 1999)—they will be able to extract more pleasure from being a therapist. Reuben Fine (1985) suggested that when practitioners say that the countertransference is unmanageable it is another way of saying that psychoanalysis is "an impossible profession" (Malcolm 1981). If therapists can acknowledge their countertransferences and accept them as part of doing therapeutic work, "it is plain that the notion of an impossible profession is just the latest in a long series of resistances to doing analysis (and psychotherapy)" (Fine 1985, p. 19).

In the chapters that follow, my colleagues and I will share our "countertransference triumphs and catastrophes" (Giovacchini 1993) with the hope that by so doing all of us will derive more pleasure from our therapeutic work and concomitantly help our patients lead more fulfilling lives.

REFERENCES

Abend, S. (1989). Countertransference and psychoanalytic technique. *Psychoanalytic Quarterly* 58:374–395.

Aron, L. (1996). *A Meeting of Minds: Mutality in Psychoanalysis.* Hillsdale, NJ: Analytic Press.

Alexander, F., and French, T. (1946). *Psychoanalytic Therapy.* New York: Ronald.

Balint, M., and Balint, A. (1939). On transference and countertransference. *International Journal of Psycho-Analysis* 20:223–230.

Brenner, C. (1985). Countertransference as compromise formation. *Psychoanalytic Quarterly* 54(2):155–163.

Breuer, J., and Freud, S. (1936). On the psychic mechanism of hysterical phenomena. *Studies on Hysteria*, pp. 1–13.

20 CONTROVERSIES ON COUNTERTRANSFERENCE

New York: Nervous and Mental Disease Publishing Company.

Deutsch, H. (1926). Occult processes occurring during psychoanalysis. In *Psychoanalysis and the Occult*, ed. G. Devereux, pp. 120–139. New York: International Universities Press, 1953.

Epstein, L., and Feiner, A. (1979). *Countertransference: The Therapist's Contribution to the Therapeutic Situation*. New York: Jason Aronson.

Feiner, A. (1977). Countertransference and the anxiety of influence. In *Countertransference: The Therapist's Contribution to the Therapeutic Situation*, ed. L. Epstein and A. Feiner, pp. 105–128. New York: Jason Aronson.

Ferenczi, S. (1919). On the technique of psycho-analysis. In *Further Contributions to the Theory and Technique of Psychoanalysis*, pp. 177–189. London: Hogarth, 1950.

———— (1932). *The Clinical Diary of Sandor Ferenczi*, trans. J. Dupont. Cambridge, MA: Harvard University Press, 1988.

Fine, R. (1985). Countertransference and the pleasures of being an analyst. *Current Issues in Psychoanalytic Practice* 2(3/4):3–20.

Fliess, R. (1953). Countertransference and counteridentification. *Journal of the American Psychoanalytic Association* 1:268–284.

Freud, S. (1910). The future prospects of psycho-analytic therapy. *Standard Edition* 11:139–152.

———— (1912a). Recommendations to physicians practising psychoanalysis. *Standard Edition* 12:111–120.

———— (1912b). The dynamics of transference. *Standard Edition* 12:97–108.

Fromm-Reichmann, F. (1950). *Principles of Intensive Psychotherapy*. Chicago: University of Chicago Press.

Giovacchini, P. (1979). Countertransference with primitive mental states. In *Countertransference: The Therapist's*

Contribution to the Therapeutic Situation, ed. L. Epstein and A. Feiner, pp. 235–266. New York: Jason Aronson.
———— (1993). *Countertransference Triumphs and Catastrophes*. Northvale, NJ: Jason Aronson.
Glover, E. (1927). Lectures on technique in psychoanalysis. *International Journal of Psycho-Analysis* 8:311–338.
Greenson, R. (1967). The "real" relationship between the patient and the psychoanalyst. In *The Unconscious Today*, ed. M. Kanzer, pp. 213–232. New York: International Universities Press.
———— (1974). Loving, hating, and indifference toward the patient. *International Review of Psycho-Analysis* 1:259–266.
Grosskurth, P. (1991). *The Secret Ring*. Reading, MA: Addison-Wesley.
Heimann, P. (1950). On countertransference. *International Journal of Psycho-Analysis* 31:81–84.
Issacharoff, A. (1976). Barriers to knowing in psychoanalysis. *Contemporary Psychoanalysis* 14: 389–422.
Issacharoff, A., and Hunt, W. (1978). Beyond countertransference. *Contemporary Psychoanalysis* 14:291–310.
Jacobs, T. (1986). On countertransference enactments. *Journal of the American Psychoanalytic Association* 43:289–307.
———— (1999). On the question of self-disclosure by the analyst: Error or advance in technique? *Psychoanalytic Quarterly* 68(2):159–183.
Jones, E. (1953). *The Life and Work of Sigmund Freud*. New York: Basic Books.
Kernberg, O. (1965). Notes on countertransference. *Journal of the American Psychoanalytic Association* 13:38–56.
Little, M. (1951). Countertransference and the patient's response to it. *International Journal of Psycho-Analysis* 38:240–254.
Low, B. (1935). The psychological compensation of the analyst. *International Journal of Psycho-Analysis* 16:1–8.

Malcolm, J. (1981). *Psychoanalysis: The Impossible Profession.* New York: Knopf.

Maroda, K. (1994). *The Power of Countertransference.* Northvale, NJ: Jason Aronson.

—— (1999). *Seduction, Surrender and Transformation: Emotional Engagement in the Analytic Process.* Hillsdale, NJ: Analytic Press.

McLaughlin, J. (1981). Transference, psychic reality and countertransference. *Psychoanalytic Quarterly* 50:639–664.

Mendelsohn, R., Bucci, W., and Chouhy, R. (1992). Transference and countertransference: a survey of attitudes. *Contemporary Psychoanalysis* 28(2):364–390.

Menninger, K. (1973). *Psychoanalytic Theory of Technique,* 2nd ed. New York: Basic Books.

Mitchell, S. (1988). *Relational Concepts in Psychoanalysis.* Cambridge, MA: Harvard University Press.

Moore, B., and Fine, B. (1990). *Psychoanalytic Terms and Concepts.* New Haven, CT: Yale University Press.

Natterson, J. (1991). *Beyond Countertransference: The Therapist's Subjectivity in the Therapeutic Process.* Northvale, NJ: Jason Aronson.

Nelson, M., Nelson, B., Sherman, M., and Strean, H. (1968). *Roles and Paradigms in Psychotherapy.* New York: Grune & Stratton.

Racker, H. (1968). *Transference and Countertransference.* New York: International Universities Press.

Reich, A. (1951). On countertransference. *International Journal of Psycho-Analysis* 32:25–31.

—— (1966). Empathy and countertransference. In *Psychoanalytic Contributions,* ed. A. Reich, pp. 344–360. New York: International Universities Press, 1973.

Renik, O. (1993a). Analytic interaction: conceptualizing technique in light of the analyst's irreducible subjectivity. *Psychoanalytic Quarterly* 62:553–571.

—— (1993b). Countertransference enactment and the psychoanalytic process. In *Psychic Structure and Psychic*

Change: Essays in Honor of Robert S. Wallerstein, M.D., ed. M. J. Horowitz, O. Kernberg, and E. Weinshel, pp. 137–160. Madison, CT: International Universities Press.

—— (1995). The ideal of the anonymous analyst and the problem of self-disclosure. *Psychoanalytic Quarterly* 64: 466–495.

—— (1999). Playing one's cards face up in analysis: an approach to the problem of self-disclosure. *Psychoanalytic Quarterly* 68:521–540.

Sandler, J. (1976). Countertransference and role responsiveness. *International Review of Psycho-Analysis* 3: 43–48.

Sandler, J., Holder, A., and Dare, C. (1970). Basic psychoanalytic concepts: countertransference. *British Journal of Psychiatry* 117:83–88.

Searles, H. (1975). The patient as therapist to his analyst. In *Tactics and Techniques in Psychoanalytic Therapy*, vol. II, ed. P. Giovacchini, pp. 95–151. New York: Jason Aronson.

—— (1987). Countertransference as a path to understanding and helping the patient. In *Countertransference: A Comprehensive View of Those Reactions of the Therapist to the Patient that May Help or Hinder Treatment*, ed. E. Slakter, pp. 131–163. Northvale, NJ: Jason Aronson.

Silverman, M. (1985). Countertransference and the myth of the perfectly analyzed analyst. *Psychoanalytic Quarterly* 54(2):175–199.

Slakter, E. (1987). *Countertransference: A Comprehensive View of Those Reactions of the Therapist to the Patient that May Help or Hinder Treatment*. Northvale, NJ: Jason Aronson.

Stern, A. (1924). On the countertransference in psychoanalysis. *Psychoanalytic Review* 2:166–174.

Stolorow, R. (1984). *Structures of Subjectivity: Explorations in Psychoanalytic Phenomenology.*. Hillsdale, NJ: Analytic Press.

Stolorow, R., and Atwood, G. (1979). *Faces in a Cloud:*

Subjectivity in Personality Theory. New York: Jason Aronson.

Strachey, J. (1934). The nature of the therapeutic action of psychoanalysis. *International Journal of Psycho-Analysis* 15:127–159.

Strean, H. (1959). The use of the patient as consultant. In *New Approaches in Child Guidance*, ed. H. Strean, pp. 53–63. Metuchen, NJ: Scarecrow Press, 1970.

—— (1970). *New Approaches in Child Guidance*. Metuchen, NJ: Scarecrow Press.

—— (1982). A note on the treatment of the schizophrenic patient. In *Controversy in Psychotherapy*, ed. H. Strean, pp. 146–153. Metuchen, NJ: Scarecrow Press.

—— (1993). *Therapists Who Have Sex With Their Patients: Treatment and Recovery*. New York: Brunner/Mazel.

Winnicott, D. (1949). Hate in the countertransference. *International Journal of Psycho-Analysis* 30:69–74.

2

Countertransference and Theoretical Predilections as Observed in Some Psychoanalytic Candidates

Although it is now accepted as an axiom of psychoanalytic practice that every aspect of the clinician's activity is a reflection of his current countertransference position, minimal consideration has been given in the literature to the relationship between the analyst's current countertransference position and his current theoretical perspective. Following a brief review of some of the pertinent literature, three case illustrations are presented that demonstrate how psychoanalytic candidates can misuse theoretical constructs to rationalize, rather than analyze, certain countertransference enactments and how their supervisors can collude with them in doing so.

One of the major advances in psychoanalytic theory and practice during the last two decades has been the broadening of our understanding and use of the concept of countertransference. From Freud's original dictum that "the countertransference arises (in the analyst) as a result of the patient's influence on his unconscious feelings, and we are almost inclined to insist that he shall recognize this countertransference in himself and overcome it" (1910, pp. 144–145), current practitioners tend to view countertransference as including "all of the emotional reactions at work" (Abend 1989, p. 374). Rather than an obstacle to be overcome, countertransference is now regarded by most dynamically oriented clinicians as "all those reactions of the analyst to the patient that may help or hinder treatment" (Slakter 1987, p. 3).

There is now a rather large psychoanalytic literature on countertransference, and most authors acknowledge that it is as ever-present as transference and must be constantly studied by all analysts, from the neophyte to the very experienced (Abend 1982, 1989, Barchilon 1958, Boesky 1990, Brenner 1985, Fine 1982, Heimann 1950, Jacobs 1986, Kernberg 1965, Little 1951, Renik 1993, Sandler 1976, Strean 1993). Virtually all authors agree that, like transference, countertransference can frequently be subtle but is always an important influence on analytic outcome. Furthermore, most writers concur that analyzing countertransference is no less difficult for the most experienced analyst than it is for the analytic candidate.

The increased examination and discussion of countertransference has helped most analysts to recognize that the psychoanalytic process is always an interactive one. Boesky stated the issue poignantly: "I consider the 'purity' of a theoretic analytic treatment, in which all of the resistances are created only by the patient, to be a fiction. If the analyst does not get emotionally involved sooner or later in a matter that he has not intended, the analysis will not proceed to a successful conclusion" (1990, p. 573). Just as there can be no analysis without constant transference reactions and resistances on the part of the patient, most current analytically oriented clinicians would contend that no analysis proceeds without constant countertransference reactions and counterresistances.

Another illuminating insight that has evolved from the

study of countertransference in greater breadth and depth is the current view that it is a central component in the analyst's use of treatment procedures. How and when the analyst is silent, poses questions, confronts, clarifies, interprets, or uses parameters is based on her countertransference at the time of the intervention. Jacobs (1986) has demonstrated that analytic technique is almost always a countertransference enactment even when the technical procedure is considered to be a valid and acceptable analytic intervention.

Perhaps one of the most valuable contributions to our current study of countertransference enactments has been made by Renik (1993). Recognizing that the analyst's individual psychology constantly determines his analytic posture, Renik has clearly demonstrated that "awareness of countertransference is always retrospective, preceded by countertransference enactment" (p. 556). Just as no analysand who is in the middle of a transference reaction is consciously aware of her distortion—does not say, for example, "I am now making you my seductive mother"—the same may be said of the analyst and his countertransference responses. It is only after the countertransference enactment that the analyst may become aware of the nature of his personal involvement.

Renik (1993), like many other authors (for example, Brenner 1985, Fine 1982, Jacobs 1986) has demonstrated that the analyst "cannot eliminate, or even diminish his or her subjectivity" (p. 562). We are always personally involved as we make professional assessments, clinical decisions, therapeutic interventions, and choices of theoretical models.

COUNTERTRANSFERENCE AND THEORETICAL ORIENTATION

Despite the tendency of contemporary analysts to believe that every aspect of an analyst's clinical activity is determined in part by her personal psychology, only limited consideration has been given in the literature to *how* the analyst's counter-transference wishes, defenses, superego admonitions, ideals, history, and so forth exert their influence on her theoretical perspective at a given time with a given analysand.

This would, however, seem to be an important issue, particularly today. Pine (1988) has demonstrated that there are at least four psychologies of psychoanalysis that form the basis of clinical work, and Pulver (1993) has suggested that a contemporary analyst influenced by so many theoretical perspectives is essentially an eclectic clinician. If analysts are indeed using several theoretical models in their clinical work, it behooves us to ask ourselves what personal investments were at work when we chose theoretical rationales for our treatment from among the concepts of mainstream Freudian analysis, self psychology, the object relations school, ego psychology, or from some other school of psychoanalytic thought such as those of Lacan or Melanie Klein.

My own interest in the relationship between counter-transference and theoretical predispositions evolved from a doctoral seminar entitled "Personality Theory and Clinical Practice," which I taught for several years. In studying the life histories of prominent personality theorists (psychoanalytic, neo-psychoanalytic, and non-psychoanalytic), the doctoral candidates and I were able to demonstrate that the source of many of the theorists' key conceptualizations could be found in their personal histories (Strean 1975). For example, as we studied the life of Karen Horney and learned that she was a lonely girl during most of her childhood, frequently lamenting that she could not travel on his voyages with her sea captain father, we were better able to appreciate her notion that all neuroses have as their major etiological source "loneliness in a hostile world." When we discovered that Alfred Adler was a short fellow who suffered from many physical diseases, we could address his notion of "organic inferiority" with more sophistication. We could also understand why he assumed that the child's ordinal position in the family was crucial in his or her development when we learned that Adler himself was the youngest child in his family and was very much scapegoated. Harry Stack Sullivan postulated that every child, in order to grow to full maturity, "needs a chum." Being a lonely, friendless boy on a farm might have stimulated Sullivan to think along these lines, just as sleeping in the parental bedroom may have aided Freud in discovering the Oedipus complex.

With sophistication and detail, Atwood and Stolorow (1984) have been able to demonstrate that the conceptual framework of psychoanalysts such as Freud, Reich, and Jung are very much related to their life stories and personal conflicts. To a lesser extent, a reader of *Psychoanalytic Pioneers* (Alexander et al. 1965) can observe some links between the pioneer's personal life and his theoretical framework. For example, Otto Rank became convinced that from birth he was destined to be miserable, and tried valiantly to separate himself from his past. His key concepts, *the birth trauma* and *separation anxiety*, probably evolved from his life story.

That psychotherapists find psychoanalytic and psychological concepts to bolster their self-esteem, reinforce defenses, preserve introjects, and placate their superegos is well documented in Burton's (1972) *Twelve Therapists*, in which therapists from various schools of psychoanalytic and psychotherapeutic thought were asked to present salient features of their autobiographies and demonstrate how crucial events and significant relationships had affected their therapeutic orientations. Without exception, all the clinicians found concepts and constructs from various theories in order to offer a rationale for their modus operandi in the clinical situation. For example, psychoanalyst Reuben Fine, who spent many years looking for love and trying to find it by working hard for long days and nights as a chess master and later as a psychologist, not surprisingly found Freud's notions on work and love very compatible with his own clinical orientation. Fine later formulated *the analytic ideal* (1982), which is a guide for practitioners in the clinical therapeutic situation, and emphasized how patients can grow from feeling loved by a disciplined therapist.

Sussman (1992) investigated the motives of individuals who became psychotherapists, as well as the gratifications and displeasures they derived from their work. Again, their theoretical predilections invariably were found to have evolved from their life experiences and internal dynamics.

In the literature that relates the clinician's theoretical orientation to his or her life history and character, it would appear that Renik's (1993), Jacobs's (1986), and Boesky's (1990) formulations are particularly applicable. Just as the use of a technical procedure, however valid and appropriate, emanates from the analyst's unconscious wishes, defenses, introjects, and superego mandates (Jacobs 1986), the same may be said about her choice of theoretical model. Often a concept may not be consciously chosen from, for example, drive theory, self psychology, ego psychology, or from the object relations perspective while the analyst is engaged in treatment. The analyst can enact her countertransference position at the time without much conscious awareness (Boesky 1990), and can then find concepts, constructs, and theories to buttress her analytic interventions. Rather than using theory as a guide, the analyst is misusing it to justify countertransference enactments.

When psychoanalytic and psychotherapeutic writers discuss their therapeutic interventions in the literature, they invariably present theoretical concepts to provide a rationale for their technical procedures, but the countertransference issues involved are rarely discussed. The following is a small selection from the psychoanalytic literature of case illustrations in which the author's therapeutic intervention is given a theoretical rationale, yet the intervention discussed could also be viewed as a countertransference enactment that needs to be better understood by the reader (and possibly by the writer, as well).

Blanck and Blanck

In a book on ego psychology by Blanck and Blanck (1974) the authors discuss a situation in which the analyst, on vacation, sent a postcard to an analysand. The writers view the postcard as a transitional object designed to help the patient cope better with her separation anxiety. The patient arrived late for her first session after the analyst's return, and the authors interpret her lateness as a sign of growing autonomy that should not be viewed as a form of resistance.

Although we can only hypothesize about the nature of the countertransference enactment in this vignette (as well as the vignettes that follow), it may be suggested that perhaps the analyst was experiencing some separation anxiety himself and had to keep in touch with the patient during his vacation in order to lessen his anxiety. It may also be conjectured that the analyst, not wanting to experience the patient's resentment and rejection for being infantilized, denied the patient's defiance by labeling it an act of autonomy.

Jacobson

Jacobson (1993) has described the case of a young woman who, following "an extensive period of productive interpretation of transference experiences . . . entered an hour with great excitement about a plan she was about to embark upon. Ignoring the self-destructive elements, she proceeded with great relish to outline how positively she viewed this disastrous plan" (p. 529). The analyst continued with the patient ten minutes past the end of the session. At the next session, referring to the analyst's exiting the hour, the patient said, "It hit me you were serious, really concerned. It's a serious business here, not a game we're fooling around with."

Jacobson concluded that the extra time given to the

patient was comfortable and reassuring to her. He states, "In Winnicott's terms (1963), she was for the moment responding to me primarily as 'an *environment* parent,' an arbiter of reality, rather than as 'an *object* parent' toward whom instinctual directions were being directed" (pp. 529–530).

Although Jacobson's use of Winnicott's concepts may be valid and appropriate, he makes no mention of what his patient's "disastrous" and "self-destructive" plan induced in him, particularly after "an extensive period of productive interpretation." Could the analyst have felt anxious as he identified with the patient's self-destructive behavior and therefore wanted to forestall it? Could the analyst have intuitively sensed that the patient's self-destructive behavior may have been an expression of a latent negative transference that he did not want consciously to confront at the time? Although the term environment parent may be appropriate, to understand the analyst–patient interaction in this case more fully the reader would need to have more data on the analyst's motives for breaking the ground rules. The reader would also be able to relate to the case more sensitively with some knowledge of how the analyst experienced the patient's self-destructive plans, particularly because they were announced immediately after the analyst's "productive" interpretative work.

Pulver

Pulver (1993) discusses the analytic treatment of a man during which the author used many different concepts from many different psychoanalytic schools. At one point in the analysis, the patient was enraged because the analyst refused to renegotiate the fee arrangement. When the patient jumped off the couch and headed toward the door, the analyst called out, "Roger, hold it! Let's talk about what's going on." The patient immediately complied, returned to the couch, and resumed talking and analyzing.

Pulver suggests that his intervention came out of his understanding of the patient's ego deficit. Rather than interpret the patient's conflict and his acting out, the analyst felt he had to offer some form of reparation to the patient because of the latter's inability to put his rageful impulses into words.

Again, the author's use of theoretical concepts may be valid and appropriate. However, the reader might want to know how the analyst felt when his patient acted upon his rage and wanted to leave the office. Was there a pleading tone in the analyst's directive as he was forced to face the possibility of the patient's hostile rejection and abandonment? Was the analyst's countertransference position correctly interpreted by the patient when he told the analyst that he was returning to the couch because the analyst looked hurt and the patient did not want to ever hurt anybody? In effect, did the patient *really* hurt the analyst and, in recognizing that he had done so, become frightened by his aggression and try to make some reparation?

All three of these examples suggest that analysts can use theoretical concepts to buttress their countertransference enactments. The theoretical concepts may well be valid and appropriate, but they can also serve to suppress the nature, specificity, and motives of countertransference enactment, which are most germane to every psychoanalytic process and interaction. This seems particularly pertinent to psychoanalytic candidates, who are constantly coping simultaneously with countertransference issues and theory.

COUNTERTRANSFERENCE ISSUES AND THE CHOICE OF THEORETICAL CONCEPTS BY PSYCHOANALYTIC CANDIDATES

In an ongoing seminar on analytic supervision (see Strean 1991) my colleagues and I found ourselves experienc-

34 CONTROVERSIES ON COUNTERTRANSFERENCE

ing a fair degree of discomfort as we shared an aspect of our supervisory work with each other. Although we all tended to feel reasonably comfortable while we focused our supervision on transference–countertransference interactions between the candidate and the patient, when the candidate had a tendency to overuse theoretical concepts to justify his interventions we acknowledged to each other a frequent feeling of being stymied by the candidate.

Our discussion revealed that the impasses that tended to develop in the supervision were overdetermined. First, in our eagerness to support our candidates in mastering theory, at times we failed to appreciate how they might misuse it to rationalize rather than analyze analytic interaction and interventions. Like parents delighted by their children's overt behavior (our candidates' mastering of theory), we were insensitive to what was transpiring below the surface. Second, very often when the patient and the candidate resisted facing certain transference–countertransference issues, we realized in retrospect that we were colluding with them by not confronting in supervision the issue or issues that sustained certain resistance–counterresistnce interactions (Strean 1991). Finally, we realized in hindsight that when the candidate was using heavy doses of theory to justify an intervention we almost always were critical of the particular intervention, but had some resistance to voicing our disapproval to the candidate. All of these countertransference issues contributed heavily to our resistance to helping the candidates face certain countertransference enactments with their patients.

The following are brief summaries of three situations that were discussed in our seminar.

Case 1

Dr. Barbara A., an advanced candidate, had been seeing Mr. Samuels, a man in his early forties, for about one year in four-times-a-week analysis. Mr. Samuels was in treatment because he could not sustain relationships with women, had intermittent potency difficulties, was frequently depressed, and was unable to move ahead in his work as a commercial artist.

During this first year of treatment Mr. Samuels formed an essentially positive transference toward Dr. A., experiencing her as a tender mother who was patient with him. He contrasted Dr. A. with his own mother whom he experienced as harsh, impatient, and demeaning. Over this first year in treatment, Mr. Samuels became less depressed, began dating women with less sexual inhibition and anxiety, and received a promotion in his work.

Although Mr. Samuels had few reactions to Dr. A.'s going on a four-week summer vacation, on resuming his analysis he initiated two routines in his sessions: at the beginning and end of each session he shook hands with Dr. A., and as he left the consultation room he blew her a kiss.

Asked by her male supervisor what she thought Mr. Samuels's handshaking and blowing kisses was about, Dr. A. had some very reasonable explanations. She recognized that the behavior became manifest after her summer vacation, suggesting that Mr. Samuels was trying to cope with his separation anxiety by becoming symbiotic with his analyst. However, the rituals continued, and Dr. A. did not subject them to investigation in the sessions with Mr. Samuels. When the supervisor asked why she did not discuss them with the patient, Dr. A. pointed out that Mr. Samuels had impoverished object relations during his entire life, was experiencing a good maternal object and a good breast in the form of Dr. A., enjoyed her empathy and attunement, and was deriving benefit from the corrective emotional experience in a holding environment.

Although the supervisor was beginning to feel that Dr. A. was subtly encouraging Mr. Samuels to maintain a regressed position in the transference and was acting out some material that would better have been analyzed instead, the supervisor was having difficulty sharing his impressions directly with Dr. A. As he reviewed the case situation in our supervisory seminar, he began to realize that he was impressed by Dr. A.'s theoretical sophistication as she discussed the case with him. He also became aware that he was overidentified with her pleasure in mothering Mr. Samuels, and that he was also vicariously enjoying Mr. Samuels's libidinal pleasure with Dr. A.

Eventually, when the supervisor could face his own counterresistances better, he asked Dr. A. what she thought would happen if the patient were told that since her vacation he had initiated two routines, handshaking and blowing kisses. Dr. A. quickly responded, with annoyance: "The patient would feel very angry and also feel very misunderstood. I'd be like his mother—cold and rejecting," she reflected.

It took nearly three months of weekly supervision (and personal analysis) before Dr. A. could accept the fact that analyzing, rather than gratifying, Mr. Samuels's wishes to shake hands and blow kisses could help him in his analysis and in his life, but she eventually moved in that direction. As she dealt more directly with her resistance to being the recipient of Mr. Samuels's rage toward the maternal introject, she became less indulgent and much more exploratory in her sessions with him. In her supervision, Dr. A. was less preoccupied with theoretical concepts, focused more on the transference–countertransference interaction, concentrated much of her attention on formulating helpful analytic interpretations, and took more notice of how her patient responded to them.

As these developments occurred Mr. Samuels was

enabled to discharge rage at Dr. A. for not being the ever-good mother he always wanted. After Dr. A. accepted the rage and helped him to mourn this loss, Mr. Samuels could initiate and sustain a warm, mutually loving, and sexually enjoyable relationship with a mature woman at his office. He also advanced in his work as an artist.

Case 2

Candidate Dr. James B.'s first case under control was Mrs. Hunt, a woman in her late thirties. Seen five times a week in analysis by Dr. B., Mrs. Hunt sought treatment because she was in the middle of an extramarital affair and did not know whether to leave her husband and marry her paramour or break up the affair and try to make her marriage work. Mrs. Hunt had been married for four years and, with the exception of her first few months of marriage, found her relationship with her husband unfulfilling, boring, and unstimulating. She had no children and was not formally employed.

During the first few months of her analysis Mrs. Hunt spent much of her time trying to get Dr. B. to advise her about her marriage and make a decision for her, and when this was not forthcoming she became very depressed and felt misunderstood, unloved, and unhelped. As she saw that her analyst did not alter his neutral stand her depression turned to anger, and on several occasions she threatened to leave treatment. During this time Dr. B. called her attention to a defensive pattern of hers, namely, leaving men when she was frustrated because she found it difficult and painful to sort out her feelings. Mrs. Hunt experienced Dr. B.'s confrontation as an expression of love, and rather quickly began to form an erotic transference toward him.

As he listened to Mrs. Hunt's wishes to make "mad,

passionate love" with him, which were accompanied by colorful and explicit sexual fantasies, Dr. B. responded either with unusually long silences or with many long, genetic interpretations. He repeatedly told her that she was turning him into the mother and/or father she had never had, and was trying to be a loved and loving daughter to him.

Although Dr. B. could acknowledge feeling turned on by Mrs. Hunt, he spent most of his supervisory time discussing the infantile nature of the patient's seductions. He talked a great deal about being alternately experienced as the esteemed oedipal father and the yearned-for preoedipal mother in the transference neurosis. He also pointed out that his genetic interpretations helped Mrs. Hunt's reality testing, judgment, impulse control, and other ego functions because she would eventually realize she was distorting Dr. B., thinking he was a possible lover, not her analyst.

In discussing the case in our supervisory seminar, Dr. B.'s supervisor shared her frustration in listening and relating to his extremely intellectual approach to treatment and supervision. Although impressed by his theoretical formulations, she was quite convinced that he was using them in part as a resistance to supervision and as a counterresistance in the analysis he was conducting.

With the aid of her colleagues the supervisor slowly realized that, in addition to being impressed by her supervisee's conceptualizations, she had been resisting helping him to face his own strong and persistent erotic fantasies about his patient. Furthermore, the supervisor eventually became aware that she was not helping Dr. B. to give his patient more opportunities to really experience her erotic fantasies in more depth and breadth. Dr. B. was either frustrating his analysand too much with long silences or interrupting her too much with long interpretations.

As the supervisor examined her own countertransferences toward Dr. B. and the patient, she realized that
the candidate–patient relationship induced a fair amount
of sexual anxiety in her. When she could face some of her
own voyeuristic and exhibitionistic wishes as well as her
erotic fantasies toward Dr. B. and Mrs. Hunt, she could
eventually confront her supervisee with some of his
counterresistances: for example, his unwillingness to be
experienced as a sexual man by his patient, his reluctance to temper his long silences, and his refusal to
monitor his genetic interpretations.

Although Dr. B. continued to use additional theoretical formulations in his supervision to rationalize his
therapeutic posture, the supervisor did not allow herself
to be as easily manipulated by him as she had been. It did
take Dr. B. several months before he could begin to
permit his patient to elaborate on her fantasies without
interrupting her, and even more time to let her make sure
of her own interpretations about why she was so ada-
mant in wanting to make Dr. B. a lover. Her own interpretations were more helpful to her than her analyst's
had been, in that she talked about needing reassurance
that she was "a real woman" (and not a man) and that
she needed to be a sexual object because she doubted her
own intellectual capacities.

As Dr. B. could feel more comfortable with his
sexual countertransference, he could help Mrs. Hunt to
be more accepting and curious about her sexual fantasies
toward him (Sigman 1985). As Dr. B.'s supervisor did not
collude with him in maintaining his counterresistances
(Teitelbaum 1990), Dr. B.'s misuse of theoretical concepts
declined and his working alliance with his patient improved considerably. The patient, after twenty months of
analysis, gave up her extramarital affair, helped her husband go into psychotherapy, found more satisfaction in
her marriage, and started graduate school in social work.

Case 3

Dr. C. was completing her analytic training and was in the terminal phase with her analysand, Ms. Freed. Ms. Freed was a single woman in her late twenties when she entered treatment and had been in analysis four times a week for almost four years. She had sought treatment because she found herself in constant power struggles— on her job as a hospital nurse, with men, and with relatives and friends. In addition, she had severe sexual inhibitions, phobias, and compulsions.

By the time Dr. C. and Ms. Freed mutually agreed on an ending date for the analysis, the patient had made several gains. Her sadomasochistic power struggles had lessened, she was enjoying men and sex much more, and there was a noticeable diminution in the severity and frequency of her neurotic symptoms.

With about two months to go before the ending date, Ms. Freed began coming to sessions late, had fewer associations, no dreams or fantasies, and said that she felt uninterested in the analysis. Ms. Freed dismissed interpretations by Dr. C. that she was having difficulty discussing how she felt about ending analysis. The more Ms. Freed dismissed interpretations and denied their content, the more Dr. C. persisted in trying to get her to acknowledge some of her feelings about ending treatment. It became a vicious cycle as a sadomasochistic power struggle ensued between analyst and patient.

The supervisor, a woman, brought the case to our supervisory group for discussion. It did not take our seminar long to help the supervisor to see that analyst and patient were both having a difficult time facing their mutual resistance in parting. Instead of mourning, they were fighting. The supervisor shared with us that during this time she had been seduced into long theoretical discussions with Dr. C. about termination, separation anxiety, and sadomasochism. She realized that she had been colluding with her supervisee for good reasons. Tearfully, the supervisor lamented, "I'm going to miss Dr. C., and instead of our talking about missing each other, and she and the patient missing each other, I've let us get sidetracked."

As could be anticipated, when the supervisor could share with Dr. C. how much she was going to miss her, Dr. C. could successfully weep and help her patient do the same. The patient could be helped to face her own mourning with more equanimity when her analyst and the latter's supervisor could do so first.

DISCUSSION

These three vignettes can illustrate several principles. The first to emerge clearly is that analytic candidates have a strong propensity for using theoretical concepts as a resistance to facing difficult countertransference feelings and enactments. When libidinal and/or aggressive feelings in their patients and/or in themselves stir up a kind of anxiety in the candidates that they have difficulty acknowledging, theoretical concepts may not be used as a guide but rather misused for defensive purposes. Advanced candidates seem to cope with difficult countertransference issues the way Anna Freud (1946) described teenagers coping with anxiety induced by sexual and aggressive impulses. They use intellectualization as a defense rather than face their anxiety and the fantasies that propel them.

In the first case, Dr. A. had a strong wish to maintain a symbiotic relationship with her patient and to avoid being a recipient of hostile feelings toward the maternal introject. Dr. B., in the second case, could not tolerate his patient's strong erotic fantasies toward him, or his toward her. Dr. C., in the third case, could not face her patient's longings to continue the analysis because she resisted facing the patient's and her own strong dependency on each other as well as their inevitable mourning reactions. In all three cases, the candidates used theoretical concepts to avoid awareness of the nature and specificity of their countertransference feelings and enactments. Further, by overusing many theoretical concepts in their conferences with their supervisors, the candidates could deflect discussion of countertransference issues. Again, like adolescents (A. Freud 1946), the candidates at times preferred to relate to their supervisors in an intellectual manner, rather than share their anxieties and countertransference problems.

The candidates' misuse of theoretical concepts as both a resistance to supervision and a counterresistance in their analytic work was reinforced by their supervisors. Seduced by their supervisees' erudition and not fully aware of their own countertransference and counterresistances, the supervisors protected themselves from focusing on real training issues by engaging in unnecessary theoretical discussions. Dr. A.'s supervisor was not aware of his fears of his supervisee's and her patient's rage, and used the theoretical discussions to ward it off. In addition, he derived too much vicarious gratification from the regressed symbiotic relationship between Dr. A. and her patient, and therefore did not help her analyze it. Dr. B.'s supervisor joined him in theoretical discussions in the supervision to ward off her own sexual attraction to her supervisee, and to his patient as well, in order to avoid facing some of her own voyeuristic and exhibitionistic fantasies. Finally, Dr. C.'s supervisor joined Dr. C. in conceptual preoccupations to ward off facing her own strong mourning and dependency feelings, and those of her supervisee and of the latter's patient.

It was not until the supervisors were helped to gain mastery over their own countertransference issues that they could help their trainees to do likewise. Only then did the defensive theoretical discussions abate.

As I suggested earlier in this article, the utilization of theory in treatment, like technique, can often be viewed as a countertransference enactment that can only be understood retrospectively (Jacobs 1986, Renik 1993). Although theory can help the analyst to anchor his observations and to explain much of the analytic data, our candidates quite frequently tended to misuse theoretical concepts to provide a rationale for many of their countertransference enactments and counterresistances.

The supervisory seminar's discussions helped us to appreciate that countertransference is ever-present in anybody and everybody, from the raw, inexperienced therapist to the very talented and experienced training analyst and control analyst. Seeing how supervisors collude with supervisees in maintaining counterresistances (Strean 1991), helps all of us to realize that "we all are more human than otherwise" (Sullivan 1953).

REFERENCES

Abend, S. (1982). Serious illness in the analyst: countertransference considerations. *Journal of the American Psychoanalytic Association* 30:365–379.

———— (1989). Countertransference and psychoanalytic technique. *Psychoanalytic Quarterly* 58:374–395.

Alexander, F., Eisenstein, V., and Grotjahn, M. (1965). *Psychoanalytic Pioneers*. New York: Basic Books.

Atwood, G., and Stolorow, R. (1984). *Structures of Subjectivity: Explorations in Psychoanalytic Phenomenology*. Hillsdale, NJ: Analytic Press.

Barchilon, J. (1958). On countertransference cures. *Journal of the American Psychoanalytic Association*. 6:222–236.

Blanck, G., and Blanck, R. (1974). *Ego Psychology: Theory and Practice*. New York: Columbia University Press.

Boesky, D. (1990). The psychoanalytic process and its components. *Psychoanalytic Quarterly* 59:550–584.

Brenner, C. (1985). Countertransference as compromise formation. *Psychoanalytic Quarterly* 54:55–163.

Burton, A. (1972). *Twelve Therapists.* San Francisco: Jossey-Bass.

Fine, R. (1982). *Healing of the Mind,* 2nd ed. New York: Free Press.

Freud, A. (1946). *The Ego and the Mechanisms of Defence.* New York: International Universities Press.

Freud, S. (1910). The future prospects of psycho-analytic therapy. *Standard Edition* 11:139–152.

Heimann, P. (1950). On countertransference. *International Journal of Psycho-Analysis* 31:81–84.

Jacobs, T. (1986). On countertransference enactments. *Journal of the American Psychoanalytic Association* 43:289–307.

Jacobson, J. (1993). Development observation, multiple models of the mind, and the therapeutic relationship in psychoanalysis. *Psychoanalytic Quarterly* 62:523–552.

Kernberg, O. (1965). Notes on countertransference. *Journal of the American Psychoanalytic Association* 13:38–56.

Little, M. (1951). Countertransference and the patient's response to it. *International Journal of Psycho-Analysis* 38:240–254.

Pine, F. (1988). The four psychologies of psychoanalysis and their place in clinical work. *Journal of the American Psychoanalytic Association* 36:571–596.

Pulver, S. (1993). The eclectic analyst, or the many roads to insight and change. *Journal of the American Psychoanalytic Association* 41:339–358.

Reich, A. (1951). On countertransference. In *Annie Reich: Psychoanalytic Contributions,* ed. A. Reich, pp. 136–154. New York: International Universities Press.

Renik, O. (1993). Analytic interaction: conceptualizing technique in light of the analyst's irreducible subjectivity. *Psychoanalytic Quarterly* 62:553–571.

Sandler, J. (1976). Countertransference and role responsiveness. *International Review of Psycho-Analysis* 3:43–48.

Sigman, M. (1985). The parallel process phenomenon in the supervisory relationship: a therapist's view. *Current Issues in Psychoanalytic Practice* 2:21–31.

Slakter, E. (1987). *Countertransference: A Comprehensive View of Those Reactions of the Therapist to the Patient that May Help or Hinder Treatment*. Northvale, NJ: Jason Aronson.

Strean, H. (1975). *Personality Theory and Social Work Practice*. Metuchen, NJ: Scarecrow Press.

——— (1991). Colluding illusions among analytic candidates, their supervisors, and their patients: a major factor in some treatment impasses. *Psychoanalytic Psychology* 8: 403–414.

——— (1993). *Resolving Counterresistances in Psychotherapy*. New York: Brunner/Mazel.

Sullivan, H. (1953). *The Interpersonal Theory of Psychiatry*. New York: Norton.

Sussman, M. (1992). *A Curious Calling: Unconscious Motivations for Practicing Psychotherapy*. Northvale, NJ: Jason Aronson.

Teitelbaum, S. (1990). Supertransference: the role of the supervisor's blind spots. *Psychoanalytic Psychology* 7(2): 243–258.

Winnicott, D. (1963). The development of the capacity for concern. In *The Maturational Processes and the Facilitating Environment: Studies in the Theory of Emotional Development*, pp. 73–82. New York: International Universities Press.

Discussion:
Countertransference:
A Universal Therapeutic
Phenomenon

Sally Barchilon

D r. Strean's paper addresses an important question that has been overlooked in the psychoanalytic literature, namely, in what ways does an analyst's countertransference affect her theoretical predilections? He then applies this question to senior analysts who describe their clinical work in the literature, and analytic candidates whose work is described by their supervisors. Dr. Strean shows us that senior analysts as well as beginners can be blind to their misuse of theory to justify their countertransference-driven interventions. He found instances where supervisors were seduced by their students' theoretical explanations and failed to recognize the use of theory both to resist the supervision and to disguise their countertransference.

I have found Dr. Strean's formulations very helpful to me in teaching and supervising analytic candidates and post-masters social work students. For years my students and I have found ourselves cringing at some clinical interactions we have read in the literature. Analysts who are leaders in our field and whose work we generally admire give occasional vignettes from their practice that impress us as completely off the mark. It is instructive to explore, as Dr. Strean does, what the possible sources of countertransfence contamination are. It reminds us that countertransference is as universal a phenomenon as transference and that no one is exempt. Following are two examples from articles I have used for teaching in recent years.

GIOVACCHINI'S NOTIONS AND EXPERIENCES (1992)

Giovacchini (1992) writes of two narcissistic women patients who insisted on being allowed to sit up. The first, whom he describes as a fragile, helpless woman, he allowed to sit up. He conceptualized this parameter as a response to her "inability to hold a mental representation of me and to maintain a synthesis of her self-representation unless I was in her visual field and she felt my attention focused on her" (p. 47). He later states that she never formed an analytic relationship; there was very little regression and few transference manifestations. She discontinued treatment after several months.

The second woman, who was imperious and manipulative, was told she must use the couch. Giovacchini is straightforward in discussing his reaction to this patient and admits that he would have felt too manipulated by her if he had allowed her to sit up. He again maintains that he was responding to her developmental level: she had been manipulated by her father and was now trying to treat her analyst the way she had been treated. Although furious at first at having to lie down, she was soon able to understand that it was helpful, and went on to make many therapeutic gains.

While Giovacchini may well have been correct in his assessment of the developmental levels of the two women, he does not make clear why he believed the first woman was so fragile. At one point he says he felt sorry for her. Is it possible that he could not take what seemed an aggressive stance with such a weak woman but actually enjoyed it with a strong one whom he could dominate? One wonders if the first woman experienced the analyst as not expecting too much from her, and protected herself from his perceived indifference by withdrawing emotionally and later by premature termination. One has the distinct impression that theory is invoked to buttress technical interventions to disguise the countertransference enactments.

KARON AND VANDENBOS'S EXPERIENCES

Karon and VandenBos discuss suicidal threats by a schizophrenic patient. The authors view such threats as a patient's way of aggressively retaliating against those who have hurt him. Their theoretical position is that the therapist should undercut this fantasy of successful retaliation by pointing out how actually happy other people will be if the patient commits suicide, or at worst they will be unhappy for only a short time. Thus Karon tells one of his patients that her suicide won't hurt her husband who wants a divorce anyway, that her parents will be glad to be rid of her, and "I'll just get another patient." The patient responds by saying that's the stupidest interpretation she ever heard.

Although we are told that this patient does not commit suicide, that doesn't seem to justify endorsing this therapeutic strategy. Instead, it would be worthwhile to consider what the therapist's countertransference might have been. Is it possible that the therapist might have experienced the threat of the patient's suicide as an abandonment or as reminiscent of some earlier loss that aroused angry feelings? This might explain what could be viewed as a sadistic response. Is it conceivable that the therapist felt his professional reputation was threatened and he reacted by diminishing the patient? There is no mention of what feelings were aroused in the therapist. Although the patient's aggression was discharged and suicide was avoided, the therapist's countertransference issues were not sufficiently considered.

TEACHING AND LEARNING COUNTERTRANSFERENCE

As I reflect on my own analytic training, I recall that there was relatively little attention paid to countertransference. As we read the literature, our focus was on trying to grasp the theory and emulate the technique. There was a respect for the authority of the analyst-authors that did not admit of their making mistakes, with a few notable exceptions. One of these was Freud's unwillingness to face his countertransference in his work with his teen-aged patient, Dora. If fault was found with an analytic writer, it was likely to be expressed as a theoretical difference. If fault was found with technique, the analyst was dismissed as non-analytic. Our own technical errors were attributed mainly to our inexperience. I believe that this orientation contributed to an atmosphere in which it was very difficult for students to discover or confront their countertransference feelings.

The climate today is far different. There has been a shift toward democratization of countertransference—everybody has it! Our students are free to detect it in even the most revered leaders and teachers of analysis. And that makes it far less traumatic to detect it in themselves.

In teaching classes or working individually with supervisees, countertransference issues come up in every setting. I would like to focus particularly on teaching in a group setting, whether it be in a class on technique or a practicum in which students present their own material. For a number of reasons, I find that discussion of countertransference issues is generally easier in a group setting. My practice is to have one student present clinical material and following that to ask the group to respond to the session in terms of how they feel about the patient and about the interaction between patient and therapist. First, I think that this allows the students to safely express their feelings from a distance. After all, they're not in the room with the patient and they can't be held responsible for making an error or having a feeling they later decide is inappropriate, so they are quite spontaneous in talking about the feelings stirred up in them. Second, there is usually a wide range of feelings presented because of the number of people involved. Therefore no one is targeted as one who has a bad idea or a wrong feeling. Also there is usually at least one person who feels the same way as the student presenting and this allows the presenter to feel less alone, especially when it comes to having to confront one's error based on the feelings that were aroused. Third, the others' reactions come without the weight of authority because, after all, the others are also students, also in a learning position. I also express my own feelings, which puts me on the same level in terms of a human reaction.

I would like to give a few examples of how the group setting is useful for beginning therapists to deal with countertransference issues:

Mr. J. is a therapist who worked in a program for gay men that offered time-limited therapy of ten sessions. The presentation was the final session of a therapy that had focused on Robert's feelings following the breakup of a love relationship. Robert began by saying that it had been a weird week. Mr. J. responded, "This, as you know, is our last session and I wonder if you have any feelings about that." Mr. J.'s rationale for introducing this topic in such an abrupt fashion was that he was afraid the patient would begin with a topic that would lead them away from feelings about termination and that the opportunity to discuss it would then be lost. Mr. J. felt that Robert would have difficulty dealing with the separation and he wanted to be in a position to help him with it.

When asked to respond to this opening, all but one

student felt that it was too abrupt a shift, that Robert's opening had not been responded to, and that he had not had the opportunity to develop it—that it may have even related to termination. Mr. J. repeated his concern that Robert had difficulty with losses and needed to be helped with this ending. I told the class a story from a beginning therapy case of mine that involved a young woman about my age toward whom I felt affection and protectiveness and with whom I identified. After I saw her for a year, a change in my job necessitated our ending. Following our final session, I watched her as she walked away and glanced back over her shoulder. I related this experience to a colleague and said, "She was really having a hard time with the termination." My wiser colleague said to me, "Who was having a hard time?"

The class laughed with some relief at this story, and I asked Mr. J. how he had been feeling about ending with his patient. He was able to say he felt sad about the ending, that it would be a loss for him. This led to a broader discussion of how hard it is when managed care or agency policy requires the termination of a treatment that is neither the patient's nor the therapist's choice. Mr. J. could then talk about his feeling that he was not doing his patient a service to end at this time; he knew Robert would have preferred to continue his treatment. It became clear to all of us as we discussed these issues that the therapist had acted on a number of unconscious feelings. Mr. J. had felt guilty about the forced termination and anxious about Robert's possible reaction. His anxiety was so acute that he had sought premature closure by jumping into the topic without heeding the time-honored practice of starting where your client is.

Mr. N. was a therapist working in the school system as a guidance counselor. His patient, Judy, was 16, from a West Indian background. Her parents had separated but had recently begun a reconciliation, which Judy was against. Her grades had precipitously dropped and she had begun cutting class. In one of their sessions, Mr. N. was listening and following along in a therapeutic manner when Judy began to express a lot of anger toward her mother and a suspicion that her mother was never really leveling with her.

At this point Mr. N. shifted his stance to one of placation. "Rome wasn't built in a day. I think you've made a lot of progress. Let's take what your mother is giving you right now, and you and I can continue to work on things you need personally that would enable you to be productive academically." The therapist described this shift as necessary because his patient was at risk of damaging her academic record, and he was needed to engage her ego to help her realistically assess what was going on at school.

The response from his fellow students was mixed. Some felt that in fact this was a difficult young woman who tended to blame others and who needed help in just focusing on the reality issues. Other students felt that Mr. N. had shifted away from trying to understand Judy and maintaining a neutral stance.

When I asked for reactions to Judy, the students said that she exuded anger. When we inquired about her immigration, we learned that Judy's parents had come ahead to the United States to establish themselves, and sent for Judy and her sister two years later. It then emerged that Mr. N. was also the son of immigrants and his history resembled Judy's. Two other students had similar histories and this led to a discussion of how abandoned the children feel when they are left behind with relatives. Mr. N. described how strange it is when you think you are going to a land of great wealth and opportunity and find that it's very cold, that you are confined to a small apartment because it's not safe to play outside, that you can't pick fruit from trees and so on. What became clear from the discussion was how Mr. N., through his focusing on the reality issues of school, was attempting to get Judy to suppress her anger at her mother because Mr. N. had not faced his own and wasn't ready to do so. He had taken what was really a defense against his own frightening rage and had raised it to an idealized theoretical position.

Numerous examples could be given of students altering their clinical work and giving theoretical grounds to justify it when under pressure from supervisors, agencies, or governmental directives. Mr. R., an able young therapist, revealed that he had taken to giving his patient, 17-year-old David, advice and encouragement about the diet to which he needed to adhere for medical reasons. He felt this intervention was necessary because of David's apparent masochism and the danger he was putting himself in medically. When Mr. R. was made aware of his failure to hear his patient's feelings of hopelessness and disgust for his body, which had deteriorated from strong and athletic to weak and impotent, Mr. R. could acknowledge that he had actually heard this communication and should have explored it. As he puzzled over this he became aware of how pressured he had felt by the physicians who were concerned about the patient's poor diet and weight loss. They had called on Mr. R. to "fix" the patient—make him compliant—and Mr. R. had unconsciously capitulated to this pressure instead of becoming the first person to try to understand David's emotional experience.

Mrs. L. also worked in an outpatient medical setting. When her patient, Ms. Y., became increasingly paranoid and belligerent toward her neighbors, she required a brief hospitalization. In their first session following the hospitalization, Mrs. L. felt the need to repeatedly remind Ms. Y. that she must be conscientious about taking her psychotropic medication to control her paranoia. Mrs. L.'s stated reason for this was that the patient was externalizing her problems and projecting her rage and needed to be reminded that it was her psychological symptoms that had necessitated the hospitalization.

While this was a valid formulation, it seemed to hide a countertransference enactment in which Mrs. L. had assumed a parental stance. When this was pointed out, Mrs. L. could focus on her feelings as a reaction to the pressure she felt from her supervisor and other medical personnel. It had happened that within the previous few months, there had been two incidents at that institution that had received prominent negative press. The atmosphere among the professional staff was one of extreme tension. Mrs. L.'s supervisor had repeatedly spoken of the risks inherent in releasing Ms. Y., and Mrs. L. was drawn into taking a stance of trying to protect her patient as well as her institution.

COMMENTS

I have taken Dr. Strean's concept of overuse of theory as a countertransference enactment and applied it to my own experience in working with a student group that is less advanced than analytic candidates. It has proven immensely helpful to this group and has allowed them to become aware of the many pressures impinging on their interventions. They have learned to question their use of theoretical arguments to support some of their interventions and thus to uncover unconscious or preconscious pressures that they have acted on in a way best described as determined by countertransference.

REFERENCES

Giovacchini, P. L. (1982). Structural progression and vicissitudes in the treatment of severely disturbed patients. In *Technical Factors in the Treatment of the Severely Disturbed Patient*, ed. P. L. Giovacchini and L. B. Boyer, pp. 3–62. New York: Jason Aronson.

Karon, B., and VandenBos, G. R. (1981). *Psychotherapy of Schizophrenia*. New York: Jason Aronson.

Discussion: Variations in the Language of Countertransference*

Michael Kasper

A number of years ago I was asked to discuss Dr. Strean's then unpublished article, "Countertransference and Theoretical Predilections as Observed in Some Psychoanalytic Candidates." The occasion was a candidate-faculty meeting and graduation at the New York Center for Psychoanalytic Training, the institute where I had trained and where Dr. Strean had once been my supervisor as well as my teacher and mentor. I remember reading the article many times, trying to decide what to say, how to respond. With each reading I became more convinced that the paper was flawed, didn't make sense. I was in a transference of sorts, based on childhood conflicts displaced onto a current father figure. Eventually I came to see that my vision was clouded by an unconscious wish to be Dr. Strean's favored son and, following that, to knock the old man off. My fantasies were stimulated by the memory of a supervisory session in which a patient I was then presenting had a dream that included one

*I would like to thank Francesca Schwartz, Ph.D., for her initial suggestions and, especially, Shana Y. Schacter, MSW, and William I. Grossman, M.D., for their generous support and help.

of Strean's sons, whom he actually knew and was jealous of. It was a parallel process.

My transference, based as it was on both libidinal and aggressive impulses was strengthened when, several weeks before the event, I was speaking on the phone with Dr. Strean and he said he hoped I would take issue with something in his paper. He said it jokingly, but meant it seriously, and followed it up by saying that if I couldn't find something I should speak with him because there were several things he could suggest. I recognized his lighthearted sentiment as permission for me to relax my superego so that I might feel free to speak my mind, but I also experienced it as a challenge. In my presentation I pointed out that his suggestion, to find fault, could be viewed as his own transference statement while my willingness to gratify his wish was the countertransference. I speculated as to what, in our individual and shared histories, might account for the enactment I felt we were engaged in. Then, having both murdered and repaired the object in short order, I made some brief remarks about the content of the paper— the parallel process among patient, candidate, and supervisor (and supervisory group seminar)—and the rationalized use of theory as an intellectual defense of unresolved countertransference.

My efforts were well received and, now, six years later, I am very happy to have the opportunity to revisit his article and present several other ideas that are suggested by the material he offers. I would like to make some observations concerning the clinical material Strean has chosen and then tie the observations to psychoanalytic supervision, education, and attitude. My aim here is to describe several other ways of viewing the data of the parallel process phenomenon. These include efforts at describing the patient's induction of the therapist's countertransference, the Kleinian understanding of projective identification, Sandler's idea of the therapist's complementary response to a role the patient needs to have filled, and the view of countertransference as an empathic response based on a briefly held identification of the analyst with the patient.

PARALLEL PROCESS

Strean understands his case examples in terms of countertransference and counterresistance, and although every analytically educated practitioner commonly understands these terms, there are other models with which to view the material. For instance, in my initial discussion of Strean's article I described the dual transferential nature of our preliminary conversations. I related to him as if he was a father I needed to win over and then get rid of. He related to me as if I was a son, potentially critical of his father. These two transferences formed the core of a three-part parallel process. In this case the presentation itself acted as the third partner but it could just as easily have been the patient I had once presented in supervision who dreamed of Dr. Strean's son. It all depends on which three variables one chooses to examine. In any event there are two transferences to start with: patient to analyst and analyst to supervisor.

The nature of the two transferences is such that the patient, by virtue of the fact that the analyst has reactions to him, has the possibility of playing a part in the analyst's relationship with the supervisor. There is always transference. Indeed, Betty Joseph (1985) defines all that happens within the analytic setting as transference. Other authors might describe transference from a historical perspective, or, more specifically, as a repetition of early object relationships. Another way of saying this is that the transference reflects an underlying unresolved conflict. If the analyst has a conflict that resonates to that of the patient it can be called a countertransference, which can be manifested as a transference to the supervisor. In either case, shared aspects of the relationship between patient and analyst can be repeated in the relationship between analyst and supervisor. Should the supervisor be conflictually susceptible the result is a parallel process.

Schacter (2000, personal communication) makes the point that in a strict sense the issue in parallel process is one of behavior, not motivation. She makes a distinction between a triad in which the patient-to-analyst transference-countertransference causes an analyst-to-supervisor transference-countertransference that is not parallel (i.e., the conflicts are not shared, but both dyads are disturbed) which she calls a *chain-reaction*. A triad in which both sets of transference-countertransference do share common conflicted feelings she labels a *true parallel process*.

An example of the former would be a situation in which a furious patient, experiencing the analyst as disapproving and judgmental, is met with the analyst's offhanded dismissal, which the analyst comes to see as a countertransference. The same analyst, feeling guilty, unsure of herself, and needy, relates to the supervisor in a passively dependent way. The supervisor, reacting to the erotically charged transference of the supervisee, feels gratifyingly needed and extends the supervisory hour uncharacteristically. In this example we see two dyads that are behaviorally reactive to transference–countertransference disturbances but that do not share the same conflicts. The process is a chain reaction, beginning with the patient's transference.

In contrast, a furious patient, experiencing the analyst as disapproving and judgmental, is met with the analyst's off-hand dismissal, which we recognize as a countertransference. The analyst, angry at being perceived this way, feels that the supervisor has done nothing helpful and goes to the next supervisory hour ready to condemn and find fault. The supervisor, feeling pushed into a defensive posture, suggests that perhaps the analyst should find someone more to his liking to continue with. Here, the two dyads are both caught in transference–countertransference enactments that are fueled by shared conflicts—a true parallel process.

Grossman (1995), in discussing the uses of theory both as a way of learning about reality and as an identification with authority, observes that the best way to understand an experience is to put it to the test of an analysis of its dynamics. Once in a while a particular theoretician captures the attention of a sizable portion of her colleagues and a new "school" is born. Then, that teacher's model of the mind, or rationale for technique, is studied, usually rigidified, and made holy. The result is a reworking, reunderstanding, or redefining of what has come before. Such is the case, I believe, with the several versions of countertransference, as they relate to parallel process, which I shall describe. I do not mean to suggest that they are all the same, only called by a different name. No, they each take up a different point; they each help clarify a different aspect of the same phenomenon. Therefore, it just seems obvious, to me, that taken together they make up a formidable arsenal with which to help understand the analytic experience. However, it also seems to me cumbersome and potentially harmful to one's accurate understanding of the material to first apply a theoretical concept to the data of observation. It should be obvious that an analysis of the data should precede its correlation to a theoretical principle. This point of view is summed up in Freud's (1915) comment:

> We have often heard it maintained that sciences should be built up on clear and sharply defined basic concepts. In actual fact no science, not even the most exact, begins with such definitions. The true beginning of scientific activity consists rather in describing phenomena and then in proceeding to group, classify and correlate them. Even at the stage of description it is not possible to avoid applying certain abstract ideas to the material in hand, ideas derived from somewhere or other but

certainly not from the new observations alone. Such
ideas—which will later become the basic concepts
of science—are still more indispensable as the material is further worked over. They must at first
necessarily possess some degree of indefiniteness;
there can be no question of any clear delimitation of
their content. So long as they remain in this condition, we come to an understanding about their
meaning by making repeated references to the material of observation from which they appear to have
been derived, but upon which, in fact, they have
been imposed. [p. 117]

An important basis of Strean's paper is taken from
several journal articles written by Boesky (1990), Jacobs
(1986), and Renik (1993). All three wrote and continue to
write extensively on countertransference enactments and
their relationship to technique and theory. They each advocate for increased awareness and use of the countertransference to understand and explain the analytic process or, at
least, elements of it. Their interest is in the analyst's subjectivity and how this subjectivity affects the process.

Grossman (1995) suggests that much of what is written
in the ever-rich analytic literature is an amplification or
enlargement of what has come before (see also Bion 1967). It
is the process that Freud described in which the material of
observation and is repeatedly referred to, is recontextualized,
as new viewers find more or different meanings in it. Furthermore, Grossman points out that definitions that aim at
classifying, codifying, and naming psychoanalytic data and/or
observations are only approximately useful, at best. He would
argue, I believe, that constant analysis of dynamics and actual
description of events, ideas, situations, fantasies, and the like,
are ultimately more satisfying and accurate, both clinically
and theoretically.

There is an expanding literature regarding parallel process (Caligor 1981, Gediman and Wolkenfeld 1980, Sachs and Shapiro 1976, Wolkenfeld 1990) and a sizable literature on supervision which does not use the phrase "parallel process" but that refers to the idea (Arlow 1963, 1985, Ekstein and Wallerstein 1958, Schlesinger 1981, Searles 1955). Additionally, all of these authors have at their disposal a number of theoretical concepts that might explain their viewpoint as it relates to the mental functioning of the participants' minds: transference, countertransference, projective identification, empathy, transient identification, and role-responsiveness, to name the major ones.

Strean makes a clear case in support of his thesis: the candidates in psychoanalytic training misused theoretical concepts both as a resistance to supervision and as a counterresistance in their analytic work, and their supervisors reinforced these tendencies. It should be clear, as well, that the misuse of theory is not a problem particular to candidates. Gediman and Wolkenfeld (1980) make the point that in a parallelism among patient, analyst, and supervisor the flow of influence is omnidirectional, meaning that the disturbed response, shared by the participants, could start from any of the three. For proof of this simply observe what happens when the supervisor (at the "top" of the patient-candidate/ analyst-supervisor triad) takes on the "middle" position (in a candidate/analyst-supervisor-supervisory seminar triad). Then, the supervisor is as challenged by her desires to be helpful and masterful as the supervisee previously was, while, on occasion, feeling confused, frustrated, and insecure. In this situation the misuse of theory is as commonplace as noted in the original triad.

The first clinical example Strean describes is of candidate Dr. A., her patient, and her male supervisor. The case material has to do with Dr. A.'s summer vacation and her patient's response to the month-long break in which he initiated two routines: at the beginning and end of each session he shook hands with Dr. A. and as he left the consultation room he blew her a kiss.

Dr. A. does not interpret the patient's actions, rationalizing her lack of intervention with theoretical concepts to support her passivity while the supervisor colludes with her based on an avoidance of his supervisee's and her patient's rage, the gratification he takes in her apparent mastery of theory, and his vicarious pleasure in the symbiosis between candidate and patient that was based on Dr. A.'s maternal wishes and her fears of the patient's hostility.

Regarding the supervisor's part in the parallel process, Searles (1955) wrote about the emphasis he placed on noticing one's own feelings: "tenderness, sympathy, resentment, rage, or whatever—in the analytic relationship" (p. 160). My reading of his paper is that, on this point, he would caution us to look not only at the classical countertransference, which would locate the source of emotion in the supervisor's repressed past but also in the therapist–patient relationship and, basically, in the patient himself. So, in the case of Dr. A. we might view both her and the supervisor's disquieting emotions as seduced or induced responses to the patient's productions without knowing whether or not they are reflections of their own subjective histories. Again, Searles doesn't advise abandoning the ship of classical countertransference, by which he means the therapist's (or supervisor's) transference to the patient (or supervisor), not the sum of all the therapist's feelings vis-à-vis the patient.

This model of looking at the parallel process comes close to the contemporary Kleinian point of view (Schafer 1994) in which the Kleinians understand much of what they feel as induced countertransferences, the result of projective identification. By this they mean that the analysand unconsciously allocates or projects into the analyst those aspects or internal objects that he needs to get rid of, or to use as a method of control, or to protect himself from intensely destructive introjects. Schafer makes the point, however, that these analysts do not blind themselves to the possibility of the analyst's own self-initiated countertransference, only that they take that aspect of analytic work as requiring no special emphasis by them.

So, for instance, not only might the contemporary Kleinians look at the parallel process in terms of each player's individual transference-countertransference but they would be particularly interested in the supervisory parallelism as a reflection of the patient's projective identification of his unconsciously troubling internal objects, desires, or affects. In Strean's example the patient feared, and was angry over, the vacation separation and had destructive wishes toward the offending analyst who represented his cold and rejecting mother. What Dr. A. felt might have been understood as the patient's projection, into her, of his symbiotic strivings and ever-present worries over abandonment. Dr. A. might have felt the patient's anger as her own and responded to this uncomfortable feeling counterphobically, by expressing an opposite response—one of loving acceptance.

Reich (1960), responding to the Kleinian position on projective identification, cautions that the assumption that what is felt by the analyst, in the present, is being transmitted by the patient obviates the entire idea of a brief identification—empathic feeling—in favor of a belief that what the analyst feels is a direct expression of the current affective state of the patient, albeit his unwanted affective state. The implication of this point of view is that room is left for a "blame the victim" attitude in which the analyst can claim no personal responsibility for his countertransference.

Sandler's (1976) use of the term *role responsiveness* is an answer to what he finds lacking in the terms *projection, externalization, projective identification,* and *putting parts of oneself into the analyst.* His complaint is that these ideas do not pay enough attention to the dynamic quality of the patient–therapist interaction. Therefore, he sees the individual feelings of the actors as responsive to a system of unconscious cues in which the analyst complies with the patient's need for a particular kind of response—a complementary one. The sadist needs a masochist; the overly anxious patient needs to be reassured.

As I understand Sandler's model and apply it to our case example, he would consider seriously the countertransference positions of both candidate and supervisor but would fix his analytic gaze on the possibility of the patient's need for the candidate/analyst to fulfill an unconscious role—that she be the maternally loving and accepting mother he never had—a role she felt compelled to comply with. This is, of course, not far from what Strean describes, except that his focus is geared more toward the individual countertransference while Sandler's is more toward the shared call and response.

In a particularly sensitive article, Michael Feldman (1993) discusses various aspects of this phenomenon from both the patient's and the analyst's perspectives. To return to the case example: I understand Feldman's view as meaning that Dr. A.'s patient might need the potential reassurance of a fantasized loving and supportive mother, one who would accept his gifts without question. In the transference relationship the patient might then fantasize the analyst warmly accepting what he brings at the beginning and end of each session: a kiss and a handshake. Based on Feldman's ideas, our understanding of the case at that point would include both the ideas of projective identification and role responsiveness. We might then see the analyst's passivity as responding to the role her patient felt the need for her to inhabit: the accepting, non-critical, loving mother. Concurrently, we might think of Dr. A.'s response as a defense of her guilt for feeling cold and uncaring, feelings put inside her via projective identification.

The last model I would like to describe makes use of the terms *identification, transient identification*, and *empathy* (Arlow 1963, Caligor 1981, Greenson 1960). Arlow makes the useful observation that in presenting material in supervision a supervisee might shift his role so that he stops reporting the data of the experience with the patient, and begins experiencing the experience of the patient. This he labels as a transient identification (but not necessarily a countertransference), which signifies an empathic response of the acting-out sort. Using this as a basis for understanding Dr. A.'s part in the analytic/supervisory experience we might see her reluctance to interpret as a change from active listener (in her role as analyst), or reporter (in her role as supervisee) to empathic experiencer, the result of a brief identification. It should be noted that in the case example of Dr. A. the material suggests a real countertransference in process. However, the benefit of this model is in its teasing-out quality. The supervisee's ability to use the supervision, with relatively little conflict, speaks to the transient nature of the identification and its less troublesome aspect. Conversely, should the supervisee feel stuck in his identification, as Dr. A. seemed to, we would be alerted to view the response as a countertransference in the classical sense.

CONCLUDING THOUGHTS

Many brilliant psychoanalytic thinkers, theoreticians, and clinicians have written about the role of supervision, and several of these are already cited in this paper. By making the observation that candidates in psychoanalytic training use and misuse theory in defense of their countertransference positions and enactments with patients, Strean lends me the opportunity to address briefly the question of supervision. How does it work and who does what?

Stone (1974) writes what I see as the majority opinion: personal analysis is the cornerstone of anyone's training but supervision is a close second. He takes a dim view of supervision as an adjunctive analysis while declaring the obvious, that on occasion a supervisor might have to point out interference when it comes from a candidate's personality.

Lesser (1984), who disagrees entirely with the traditional distinctions between the psychoanalytic and supervisory situations, takes an antithetical position. She would examine the supervisee's countertransference, in depth, as it came up during supervision. As for the parallel process, Lesser seems to favor Gediman and Wolkenfeld's (1980) approach: that the locus of initiating responsibility can rest with any of the participants.

Schafer (1983) paints a broader picture when he says, "one is, in fact, always becoming an analyst" (p. 282). He joins the arguments between those who maintain strict boundaries between therapist and supervisor and those who come close to dissolving the boundaries between personal analysis and supervision. In the transcript of a live supervisory session followed by discussion (1981) he elaborates further; he tends not to discuss the content of countertransference very far with supervisees, especially if they are already in treatment. However, he will, on occasion, especially if he feels he must. He points out that there is always transference in supervision (meaning from supervisee to supervisor although, of course, the flow can be reversed). But unless it becomes disturbing to the process he doesn't feel the need to take it up.

My own experience, both as supervisee and supervisor, is similar to the models presented by Stone and Schafer. When common sense prevails, boundaries are maintained. However, in the real world the supervisor's job is to consult and teach, and sometimes this may include a deeper discussion of a supervisee's countertransference.

I have gone into this background only because Dr. Strean's article does not specify what exactly was said in order to resolve the patient-candidate-supervisor enactments—only that successful supervisory analysis (in the context of a supervisory group studying the supervisory process) helped turn things around. The point is that *something* turned things around and *some* method of understanding the interactions was employed. It would have been instructive, for the purposes of this paper, to have heard how deeply the supervisor took up Dr. A.'s, and his own, subjective responses in the actual supervisory hour. One's decison as to which model to employ to understand countertransference reaction is often based on a host of factors: where training was completed, by whom, how high up the professional ladder this person was and how much authority he carried—not to mention personal dynamics and history.

Interestingly, though, the resolution of the countertransference, parallel or not, rests on an objective outcome of a wholly subjective state. Grossman (1982), Fliess (1942), and Schafer (1983) all make similar or related points when they describe the analyst's work ego (Fliess) as a kind of second self (Schafer). Grossman describes it as the analyst's (or supervisor's) requirement to forge a unified understanding of both the patient's and his own subjective reactions—an objective view—which he calls *psychoanalytic neutrality.*

My own view is that seeing the ubiquity of the parallel process phenomenon is a little like looking for the bogey man under every cover. Parallel process, whether inevitable, as Gediman and Wolkenfeld suggest, or situational and more circumscribed, necessitates a resolution whenever it becomes apparent, one that is useful to furthering the supervision and ultimately the analysis. In this way it is no more, or less, than any piece of analytic material to be understood. A more interesting question has to do with the *way* in which we understand analytic material, our own as well as our patients', and depends on a choice we make based on factors other than "truth" and correctness. The fact that we make a choice bears directly on the fact that a choice exists. As with all questions of comparative analytic technique derived from theory, the question is: To what extent do differing models of the mind produce similar or varying analyses given the same material?

There are several models with which to view countertransference, in all their subtle and not-so-subtle complexities, and these must leave us, once and for all, with the idea

68   CONTROVERSIES ON COUNTERTRANSFERENCE

that it is only through thorough analysis of motivation, fantasy, wish, and constraint that the "truth" of a particular enactment can be made known and understood.

REFERENCES

Arlow, J. A. (1963). The supervisory situation. *Journal of the American Psychoanalytic Association* 11:576–594.
——— (1985). Some technical problems of countertransference. *Psychoanalytic Quarterly* 54(2):164–174.
Bion, W. R. (1967). *Second Thoughts: Selected Papers on Psychoanalysis*. New York: Jason Aronson.
Boesky, D. (1990). The psychoanalytic process and its components. *Psychoanalytic Quarterly* 59:550–584.
Caligor, L. (1981). Parallel and reciprocal processes in psychoanalytic supervison. *Contemporary Psychoanalysis* 17(1): 1–27.
Ekstein, R., and Wallerstein, R. S. (1958). *The Teaching and Learning of Psychotherapy*. New York: Basic Books.
Feldman, M. (1993). The dynamics of reassurance. *International Journal of Psycho-Analysis* 74:275–285.
Fliess, R. (1942). The metapsychology of the analyst. *Psychoanalytic Quarterly* 11:211–227.
Freud, S. (1915). Instincts and their vicissitudes. *Standard Edition* 14:117–138.
Gediman, H. K., and Wolkenfeld, F. (1980). The parallelism phenomenon in psychoanalysis and supervision: its reconsideration as a triadic system. *Psychoanalytic Quarterly* 49:234–255.
Greenson, R. (1960). Empathy and its vicissitudes. *International Journal of Psycho-Analysis* 41:418–424.
Grossman, W. I. (1982). The self as fantasy: fantasy as theory. *Journal of the American Psychoanalytic Association* 30: 919–937.
——— (1995). Psychological vicissitudes of theory in clinical

work. *International Journal of Psycho-Analysis* 76:885–899.

Jacobs, T. (1986). On countertransference enactments. *Journal of the American Psychoanalytic Association* 43:289–307.

Joseph, B. (1985). Transference: the total situation. *International Journal of Psycho-Analysis* 66:447–454.

Lesser, R. (1984). Supervison, illusions, anxieties, and questions. In *Clinical Perspectives on the Supervision of Psychoanalysis and Psychotherapy*, ed. L. Caligor, P. M. Bromberg, and J. D. Meltzer, pp. 143–152. New York: Plenum.

Reich, A. (1960). Further remarks on countertransference. *International Journal of Psycho-Analysis* 41:389–395.

Renik, O. (1993). Analytic interaction: conceptualizing technique in light of the analyst's irreducible subjectivity. *Psychoanalytic Quarterly* 62:553–571.

Sachs, D. M., and Shapiro, S. H. (1976) On parallel processes in therapy and teaching. *Psychoanalyic Quarterly* 45:394–415.

Sandler, J. (1976). Countertransference and role responsiveness. *International Review of Psycho-Analysis* 3:43–48.

Schafer, R. (1981). Supervisory session with discussion. In *Clinical Perspectives on the Supervision of Psychoanalysis and Psychotherapy*, ed. L. Caligor, P. M. Bromberg, and J. D. Meltzer, pp. 207–230. New York: Plenum, 1984.

——— (1983). *The Analytic Attitude*. New York: Basic Books.

——— (1994). The contemporary Kleinians of London. *Psychoanalytic Quarterly* 63:409–432.

Schlesinger, H. J. (1981). General principles of psychoanalytic supervision. In *Becoming a Psychoanalyst: A Study of Psychoanalytic Supervision*, ed. R. S. Wallerstein, pp. 29–38. New York: International Universities Press.

Searles, H. (1955). The informational value of the supervisor's emotional experience. In *Collected Papers on Schizophre-*

nia and Related Subjects, pp. 157–176. New York: International Universities Press, 1965.

Stone, L. (1974). The assessment of students' progress. In *Transference and Its Context*, pp. 367–381. Northvale, NJ: Jason Aronson, 1984.

Wolkenfeld, F. (1990). The parallel process phenomenon revisited: some additional thoughts about the supervisory process. In *Psychoanalytic Approaches to Supervision*, ed. R. C. Lane, pp. 95–109. New York: Brunner/Mazel.

3

Colluding Illusions among Analytic Candidates, Their Supervisors, and Their Patients: A Major Factor in Some Treatment Impasses

In "The Future of an Illusion," Freud (1927) averred that no man or woman has a "love for instinctual renunciation" and neither can easily "be convinced by argument of its inevitability" (p. 7). Yet, Freud also pointed out in the same work that "every civilization must be built up on coercion and renunciation of instinct" (p. 7). This notion was and continues to be an important axiom in psychoanalysis, particularly in the treatment situation wherein the analysand is helped to master her id impulses rather than "giving free rein to their indiscipline" (Freud 1927, pp. 7–8). Many, if not most, analysts have concurred with Freud's (1923) terse prescription that where there is id, there shall be ego.

Freud also suggested in "The Future of an Illusion" that "It is only through the influence of individuals who can set an example and whom masses recognize as their leaders that they can be induced to perform the work and undergo the

renunciations on which the existence of civilization depends"
(p. 8).

Though Freud did not explicitly refer to psychoanalysts
as the leaders, the implication seems to be there when he says,
"All is well if these leaders are persons who possess superior
insight into the necessities of life and who have risen to the
height of mastering their own instinctual wishes" (p. 8).

Rather early in his career, Freud recognized that if
analysts did not master their own id wishes, monitor their
own fantasies, and calm their own illusions, they could not
help their patients to do the same. Freud advised psychoanalysts to model themselves after the surgeon who puts aside all
feelings, even his human sympathy, and concentrates his
mental forces on performing the operation as skillfully as
possible. He never abandoned the paradigm of the abstinent,
anonymous surgeon (Freud 1912, 1915, 1919).

Just as the masses need leaders "who possess superior
insight into the necessities of life and who have risen to the
height of mastering their own instinctual wishes," analysands
seem to need the same from their analysts. As a matter of fact,
as early as 1910, Freud pointed out that if the analyst has not
resolved the conflicts that his patient is confronting, the
analysis will be unsuccessful. Freud said:

> We have noticed that no psycho-analyst goes further
> than his own complexes and internal resistances
> permit; and we consequently require that he shall
> begin his activity with a self-analysis and continu-
> ally carry it deeper while he is making his observa-
> tions on his patients. Anyone who fails to produce
> results in a self-analysis of this kind may at once give
> up any idea of being able to treat patients by
> analysis. [p. 145]

As we know, Freud modified his position about self-
analysis and recognized that it was very difficult to be analyst

and analysand simultaneously. Contemporary analysts often joke about this issue and say, "Self-analysis is impossible because the countertransference gets in the way!"

Actually, in contrast to his comprehensive and meticulous discussions of transference (1912, 1914, 1915, 1926), Freud wrote very little on the subject of countertransference. He did point out that "the countertransference arises [in the analyst] as a result of the patient's influence on his unconscious feelings, and we are almost inclined to insist that he shall recognize this countertransference in himself and overcome it" (1910, pp. 144–145). As Abend (1989) pointed out, "Freud's original idea that countertransference means unconscious interference with an analyst's ability to understand patients has been broadened during the past forty years: current usage often includes all of the emotional reactions at work" (p. 374). This view has received much support in the psychoanalytic literature. Slakter (1987) referred to countertransference as "all those reactions of the analyst to the patient that may help or hinder treatment" (p. 3). And, it should be mentioned that as early as 1950 Heimann referred to countertransferences as "all the feelings which the analyst experiences toward his patient" (p. 81).

Rather than viewing it as a periodic unconscious interference, there is now a rather large psychoanalytic literature on countertransference, with most authors acknowledging that it is as ever-present as transference and must be constantly studied by all analysts, from the neophyte to the very experienced (Abend 1982, 1989, Barchilon 1958, Brenner 1985, Fine 1982, Heimann 1950, Kernberg 1965, Little 1951, Reich 1951, Sandler 1976, Strean 1988). Virtually all authors agree that like transference, countertransference can frequently be subtle but is always very influential on analytic outcome. Furthermore, most writers concur that analyzing countertransference is no less difficult for the most experienced analyst than it is for the analytic candidate. Both are too easily satisfied with what Freud called "a part explanation."

Although psychoanalysts have to cope with different countertransference issues at different times, depending not only on the patient's productions, but also on the analyst's particular stage of life, current level of training and experience, and the current stresses in his life, no analyst in working with patients is exempt from experiencing childish fantasies toward them, assuming defensive postures with them, or making therapeutic interventions that emanate more from the analyst's own anxiety, disturbing memories, or superego injunctions than exclusively from the patient's associations. All analysts, like all patients, "are more human than otherwise" (Sullivan 1953).

If all psychoanalysts experience and reexperience conflicts in their work, one place where the senior analyst will be very prone to countertransference problems is in the supervisory situation. Often the supervisor or control analyst assumes this role when her own children have left home, and therefore it is a time when she is experiencing loss and often yearns to be a parent again. Consequently, many supervisors may unconsciously want to use the analytic candidate in the service of buttressing lowered self-esteem, refueling lost narcissism, or finding a lost child. Assuming a supervisory position is quite similar in many respects to becoming a parent. Therefore, the supervisor inevitably has to cope with old and new conflicts that emerge or reemerge from old and new parent–child relationships.

However, just as psychoanalysts had little to say about countertransference issues until late in psychoanalysis's history, the same can be said about the supervisor's countertransference reactions in the teaching–learning situation. For many decades psychoanalytic supervision was conceived as an arrangement in which the more experienced and more knowledgeable analyst helped the inexperienced and less knowledgeable candidate better understand the patient's dynamics, history, and transference reactions, as well as the candidate's countertransference responses, particularly how the latter colluded with his patient to avoid analyzing material that induced anxiety in the candidate and in the patient (Ekstein and Wallerstein 1972, Fleming and Benedek 1966). Very little consideration has been given to supervisors' anxieties, fantasies, and inappropriate expectations, what Teitelbaum (1990) aptly referred to as *supertransference*. How the illusions of supervisor, candidate, and patient can parallel each other to create a therapeutic impasse has been essentially overlooked.

Although as early as 1954, Benedek called attention to the importance of unresolved problems in the supervisor as a factor contributing toward negative therapeutic outcomes, twenty-five years later Langs (1979) concluded: "There has been a rather striking neglect in the literature of the supervisor's countertransferences and . . . they deserve systematic consideration" (p. 333). Later, Schlesinger (1981) echoed the same sentiment and suggested that the supervisor may unwittingly contribute to the candidate's learning problems and the patient's eventual lack of progress in treatment. In 1984 Issacharoff dealt somewhat more directly with the supervisor's countertransference issues, pointing out how she may enact a role of either overprotective parent and/or one of overly critical parent. The candidate, treated like a weak and/or disappointing son or daughter, may then act out with the patient, in the therapy, the anger and discomfort stimulated in supervision.

Just as more analytic patients and analysts have the potential to collude with each other to gratify certain illusions of the patient, such as the latter's yearning to be the analyst's favorite child, or to symbiose with the analyst and become omnipotent like the analyst appears to be, similar illusions can be present in the teaching–learning situation in which supervisor and supervisee can also collude. Supervisor and supervisee can share the illusion that the supervisor is omniscient, whereas the candidate and patient know next to nothing. They can suffer together from the illusion that the supervisor is exempt from pathology, ignorance, and blind spots, whereas the candidate and the analysand are both struggling to maintain their sanity. The learner and his mentor can delude themselves into believing that the supervisor's sexual and aggressive fantasies are in superb control whereas the patient and the analytic candidate are either too inhibited by their punitive superegos or too expressive because of their superego lacunae.

As Lesser (1984) noted, certain illusions may exist in supervision such as "the supervisor is always objective" or "the supervisor always knows best." She further pointed out that the supervisor's anxieties are "generally unrecognized, perhaps because anxieties are less acceptable to the supervisor than to [the candidate. Yet], awareness of the supervisor's anxieties is essential for fulfilling the supervisory task" (p. 147).

In the literature on supervision, a phenomenon known as *the parallel process in supervision* has been noted quite frequently (Doehrman 1976, Sigman 1985). What is meant here is that the supervisee reenacts in the supervision what the patient is doing in the therapy with the candidate. What has not been discussed in the literature to any appreciable extent is how the supervisor colludes with the supervisee to aid and abet the parallel process.

In a workshop on psychoanalytic supervision, my colleagues and I became increasingly aware of the fact that when the analytic candidate and the patient were colluding with each other to avoid exploring and confronting certain issues, quite frequently the supervisor was overtly and/or covertly contributing to the impasse as well. We found that not only was the candidate unaware of certain transference and countertransference problems in the analytic relationship, but in several instances the supervisor was both blind to these same issues and unaware of her own countertransference reactions, that is, supertransference reactions, to the candidate and/or to the patient.

Following are some examples of how the supervisor's unmastered conflicts parallel the patient's and the candidate's to create analytic impasses. In examining these case illustrations, my theoretical perspective is classical Freudian analysis. Clinicians who subscribe to a self psychology orientation or who emphasize object relations might stress different issues, highlight different themes, or have different interpretations from those I have made. However, I am hopeful that the interactive focus among patient, supervisor, and candidate will be of interest to the reader, regardless of his or her theoretical perspective.

CASE 1

Ms. A., a woman in her late twenties, had been in analysis for a year with Dr. Z., an advanced candidate in his late thirties. Ms. A. was in analysis because of depression, sexual inhibitions, and an inability to relate warmly to her boyfriend, Jack, with whom she had been living for about two years. Jack and Ms. A. had frequent and intense arguments in which they often physically hit each other.

For the first seven months of her analysis, Ms. A. made steady progress. She formed a strong positive transference to Dr. Z., which led to an ebbing of her depression, an increase in her self-esteem, and more acceptance of her sexual fantasies. As she could tolerate some of her erotic fantasies toward Dr. Z., her sexual inhibitions lessened and she had more energy available for her love life and for her work as an editor.

During the first seven months of treatment, Dr. Z. frequently thanked his supervisor for his excellent supervision, and the supervisor often lauded Dr. Z. for his ability to learn. Both supervisor and supervisee also concurred frequently on Ms. A.'s excellent talents as an analysand and constantly agreed that she used her four sessions a week quite productively.

As the mutual admiration society between Dr. Z. and his supervisor grew, with both of them increasingly pleased with Ms. A. and her analytic progress, Ms. A. grew increasingly dissatisfied with her relationship with Jack. There were many more arguments between them and their sexual relationship, which had improved, began to deteriorate. At first, Dr. Z. and his supervisor attributed the increase in the relationship's disequilibrium to Jack and his inability to adapt to Ms. A.'s therapeutic gains and increased maturity. However, as our workshop began to take note of the enormous difference between Ms. A.'s strong positive analytic transference and her strong negative reactions to Jack, it began to occur to the supervisor that Dr. Z. had been conducting himself in such a manner that Ms. A. could not feel comfortable discharging negative feelings and hostile fantasies toward Dr. Z.

As the supervisor further discussed the Ms. A.–Dr. Z. case in our workshop, it eventually became quite clear to the workshop members that the supervisor was so busy praising his student and receiving praise from him that much teaching and learning was being avoided. When the supervisor was able to accept his peers' criticisms and counsel, he was able to help Dr. Z. assist Ms. A. to get in touch with some of her hostile fantasies toward her analyst. As the collusion among the candidate, patient, and supervisor dissipated, Ms. A. began to feel warmer and more sexual toward Jack and became much less idealizing of Dr. Z.

The case of Dr. Z. and Ms. A. is not an uncommon one in analytic institutes. Over the years, many writers have argued that one of the impediments to helping practitioners mature to their optimum is the nature of psychoanalytic training programs, which tend to foster too much childish dependency in their candidates and provide too much infantile gratification for them. Arlow (1982) suggested that much of psychoanalytic education inadvertently tends to further the candidates' desire to overcome their difficulties by identifying themselves with their own analyst. Furthermore, this tends to be reinforced by the idealization of authority figures, which interferes with the candidates' movement in their personal analyses and with their professional growth. The training, therefore, may not work through the candidates' identifications, with a concomitant lack of development of insight; instead, little is resolved and only the identification takes place. Arlow also commented on the curricula used in most institutes, which encourage imitation of the master rather than independent and critical examination of the data.

CASE 2

Patient, candidate, and supervisor very often maintain an unconscious symbiotic collusion. This is demonstrated quite clearly in the following case.

Mr. B., a 24-year-old, single graduate student, was in psychoanalytic treatment with Dr. V., an analytic candidate in her late thirties who was just beginning to do control analysis. Mr. B. was her first analytic case.

The patient was being seen in analysis because he was doing poor academic work in graduate school. Prior to beginning treatment, he had been doing good work but as he neared completion of his studies and was beginning to consider writing a dissertation, he lost enthusiasm for his work, suffered from insomnia, felt quite depressed, and had very little interest in people.

After about nine months of four-times-a-week analysis, Mr. B., who had been a very cooperative patient, began to question the value of the treatment. Although he acknowledged that Dr. V. had been helpful to him in lessening his depression and assisting him to develop more motivation to do work in his studies, he wondered about her as a human being. He began to experience Dr. V. as cold, detached, and emotionally unavailable. He also began to question Dr. V.'s credentials and felt that maybe she was too young and too inexperienced to do this work. He further pointed out that he felt "very much alone here—as if you are not in the room."

From the patient's history of being strongly attached to a very engulfing mother who severely controlled him and whom he described as overeager and overzealous, Dr. V. was able to grasp the idea that her analysand was defending powerfully against wishes to merge with her by becoming detached and negativistic. She was also able to see that some of Mr. B.'s negativism in the transference mirrored his negativism in his graduate studies. However, Dr. V. felt helpless in analyzing Mr. B.'s negative transference with him. She found herself tongue-tied and could not feel comfortable verbalizing inter-pretations and confrontations agreed upon in supervisory conferences. Furthermore, when Mr. B. would repeatedly fire questions at her, she felt like placating him by answering him, knowing this would not be helpful, and then giving him half-hearted interpretations that he was avoiding looking at what he felt by asking a lot of questions.

When the supervisor pointed out to Dr. V. that she appeared very intimidated, angry, and impotent with her patient, Dr. V. rather quickly withdrew from the supervisor and had almost nothing to do with him in the next several supervisory sessions. On the supervisor's commenting about Dr. V.'s withdrawal, the candidate appeared very reluctant to discuss anything with him. Instead, like Mr. B. in the therapy, Dr. V. began to ask many theoretical and technical questions in supervision about merging and symbiotic longings, and expressed her doubts about whether early preoedipal prob-lems can ever be resolved by an analysis.

On discussing Dr. V. and her patient in our workshop, the supervisor slowly realized that he was helping to recapitulate with Dr. V. in supervision what Dr. V. was doing in the treatment. Just as Mr. B. felt unhelped by Dr. V., and therefore was not examining himself, Dr. V. was doing the same in supervision. As the supervisor discussed with his colleagues how both Dr. V. and her patient appeared discouraged, disappointed, and despondent, it occurred to him that Dr. V. reminded him of his daughter who had recently gone out of town to college. Speaking of Dr. V., the supervisor said, "I'd like to take her in my arms as if she were my own daughter and say, 'Everything will be all right.' Instead, I'm acting too proper and too stiff and damn it, that's what she's doing with her patient."

As the supervisor felt understood and accepted by his peers in the supervisory seminar, he could become more sensitive to Dr. V.'s difficulties. Instead of trying to answer her questions or mechanically throw them back to her (as Dr. V. was doing with Mr. B.), the supervisor suggested to Dr. V. that from a position of feeling quite optimistic about what psychoanalysis could offer, she had become very doubtful. From conversing easily and spontaneously with the supervisor, she was asking many questions. He suggested, "Perhaps we can figure out together what's happening between us—then maybe it will be easier to see what's going on in the treatment."

Dr. V. thought a great deal about the question posed to her. She then pointed out, "Obviously we [Mr. B. and Dr. V.] are both avoiding each other! I wonder what we are avoiding." Here, the supervisor recalled an earlier discussion from supervision and reminded Dr. V. that she had been able to formulate quite clearly that Mr. B. was resisting facing his symbiotic longings in the transference. Dr. V. responded to the supervisor's reminder with enormous gratitude and intense affect, saying, "I would not have thought of that in years!" With tears she said, "I feel embarrassed to tell you how close I feel to you and how highly I regard you!" Slowly, Dr. V. was able to share with her supervisor her strong desire to have "a feeding mother," how difficult this was to face in her own analysis, and how much she would love to be that mother for Mr. B.

As Dr. V. could face her own symbiotic wishes in her

supervisory relationship, she could more easily accept her desire to be the preoedipal mother for Mr. B. and help him confront his deep desire to have Dr. V. infantilize him the way his own mother had done. To help Dr. V. do this, the supervisor first had to face his own symbiotic longings for his daughter. When he was not feeling so defended, he could be a more enabling figure for Dr. V., who could then be the same for Mr. B.

In the case of Mr. B., Dr. V., and the supervisor, all three individuals were protecting themselves and each other against symbiotic yearnings. It was not until the supervisor could resolve some of his own resistances toward his symbiotic yearnings for his daughter that the supervision and the therapy could move in a productive fashion.

CASE 3

Dr. W., an advanced candidate in her forties, was working on her last analytic case as a student. Her patient, Ms. C., a single woman in her early thirties, had been in analysis four times a week for approximately two years, having come into treatment with many presenting problems. She could never complete a task in her work as a computer specialist, feared involvement, particularly with men, and was extremely frightened of sex. She had numerous psychosomatic complaints—stomachaches, headaches, heart palpitations, and insomnia.

In the two years she had been in analysis, Ms. C. has made limited progress. Though her psychosomatic problems diminished somewhat and her work habits improved a little, her fears of intimacy, commitment, and sexuality did not abate very much. Throughout the two years of treatment, the patient had a great deal of difficulty facing and discussing transference reactions—positive and negative—and did not really form any intimate relationships on the outside.

During the third year of treatment, Ms. C. was offered a

job several thousand miles away from where the analysis was being conducted. She told her analyst that inasmuch as she was "cured," she planned to end the analysis and take the job.

When Dr. W. discussed the suggested termination in supervision, it was clear that she was not too distressed about Ms. C. leaving treatment. The more the supervisor wondered about this, the less Dr. W. related to the topic. Instead, she questioned whether Ms. C. was a good analytic case that needed analytic supervision.

As the supervisor discussed the Dr. W.–Ms. C. case with his peers, he realized that he was harboring a great deal of hostility toward Dr. W. She reminded him of his daughter-in-law "who took my son away." Further, the supervisor felt very protective of Ms. C., as if she were a daughter or son who was being mistreated. However, the supervisor was not conscious of his resentments until he presented the case situation to his colleagues. He realized through his discussion with them that by not facing his resentment toward his supervisee and his overprotective reaction toward his patient, he was colluding in the maintenance of a mutual defense among all parties that kept hostility from emerging.

After presenting the case in the workshop, the supervisor was able to suggest empathetically to Dr. W. that both she and the patient seemed to want to get away from each other. Dr. W., for the first time in supervision, became very animated and expressed a great deal of anger toward the supervisor and the analytic institute for not being more emotionally available to her. She felt that she was always so much on her own. Dr. W., who was usually mild and deferential, began to become more expressive and assertive. As the supervisor was able to face his rage toward Dr. W., Dr. W. could face her rage toward her patient and was eventually able to get in tune with Ms. C.'s rage toward her.

As it turned out, supervisor, patient, and candidate were in an intense collusion, all defending themselves and each other against destructive fantasies by a superficial blandness.

CONCLUSION

Several writers have discussed the fact that all analytic patients have secrets that they do not wish to reveal to their analysts (Fine 1982, Strean 1984). What has not been acknowledged sufficiently is that analyst and analytic supervisors also try to maintain secrets. Frequently, patient, analyst, and supervisor, as the cases discussed here were intended to demonstrate, are all colluding in maintaining a similar secret. Jacobs (1989) focused on an aspect of the transference neurosis that is frequently not recognized because it is concealed beneath the surface material. This overt dimension is related "to secrets that have played important roles in the lives of both patient and analyst" (p. 515). Jacobs also commented on the frequency "with which collusions between patient and analyst occur in the analytic situation. Such collusions, which reflect the need on the part of both participants to guard secrets of their own, may result in the failure to explore an important aspect of the transference neurosis" (pp. 515–516).

What can be added to Jacobs's assessment is that by guarding secrets of her own, the supervisor (as noted in the cases in this article) helps the supervisee and the supervisee's patient to guard and maintain secrets similar to those the supervisor is trying to keep from consciousness.

Unconscious collusion among patient, candidate, and supervisor may be viewed in terms of what Sandler (1976) called *role responsiveness*. Patient, analyst, and supervisor abdicate their assigned roles and adapt to each other's unconscious role assignments. This form of role reciprocity maintains the analysis but does not help it progress. However, as has been demonstrated, if the supervisor becomes aware of her role in the collusion, the treatment situation seems to improve markedly for both the analytic candidate and the patient.

REFERENCES

Abend, S. M. (1982). Serious illness in the analyst: counter-transference considerations. *Journal of the American Psychoanalytic Association* 30:365–379.

———— (1989). Countertransference and psychoanalytic technique. *Psychoanalytic Quarterly* 58:374–393.

Arlow, J. (1982). Psychoanalytic education: a psychoanalytic perspective. *Annual of Psychoanalysis* 10:5–20.

Barchilon, J. (1958). On countertransference cures. *Journal of the American Psychoanalytic Association* 6:222–236.

Benedek, T. (1954). Countertransference in the training analyst. *Bulletin of the Menninger Clinic* 18:12–16.

Brenner, C. (1985). Countertransference as compromise formation. *Psychoanalytic Quarterly* 54(2):155–163.

Doehrman, M. J. (1976). Parallel processes in supervision and psychotherapy. *Bulletin of the Menninger Clinic* 40:9–84.

Ekstein, R., and Wallerstein, R. S. (1972). *The Teaching and Learning of Psychotherapy*. New York: International Universities Press.

Fine, R. (1982). *The Healing of the Mind*, 2nd ed. New York: Free Press.

Fleming, J., and Benedek, T. (1966). *Psychoanalytic Supervision*. New York: Grune & Stratton.

Freud, S. (1910). The future prospects of psycho-analytic therapy. *Standard Edition* 44:141–151.

———— (1912). The dynamics of transference. *Standard Edition* 12:99–108.

———— (1914). Remembering, repeating and working-through. *Standard Edition* 12:147–156.

———— (1915). Observations on transference-love. *Standard Edition* 12:159–173.

———— (1919). Lines of advance in psychoanalytic therapy. *Standard Edition* 17:159–168.

———— (1923). The ego and the id. *Standard Edition* 19:12–68.

—— (1926). Inhibitions, symptoms and anxiety. *Standard Edition* 20:77–175.

—— (1927). The future of an illusion. *Standard Edition* 21:3–56.

Heimann, P. (1950). On countertransference. *International Journal of Psycho-Analysis* 31:81–84.

Issacharoff, A. (1984). Countertransference in supervision: therapeutic consequences for the supervisee. In *Clinical Perspectives on the Supervision of Psychoanalysis and Psychotherapy*, ed. L. Caligor, P. M. Bromberg, and J. D. Meltzer, pp. 89–104. New York: Plenum.

Jacobs, T. (1989). Notes on the unknowable: analytic secrets and the transference neurosis. *Psychoanalytic Quarterly* 58:515–516.

Kernberg, O. (1965). Notes on countertransference. *Journal of the American Psychoanalytic Association* 13:38–56.

Langs, R. (1979). *The Supervisory Experience*. New York: Jason Aronson.

Lesser, R. (1984). Supervision, illusions, anxieties, and questions. In *Clinical Perspectives on the Supervision·of Psychoanalysis and Psychotherapy*, ed. L. Caligor, P. M. Bromberg, and J. D. Meltzer, pp. 143–152. New York: Plenum.

Little, M. (1951). Countertransference and the patient's response to it. *International Journal of Psycho-Analysis* 38:240–254.

Reich, A. (1951). On countertransference. In *Annie Reich: Psychoanalytic Contributions*, pp. 136–154. New York: International Universities Press.

Sandler, J. (1976). Countertransference and role responsiveness. *International Review of Psycho-Analysis* 3:43–48.

Schlesinger, H. (1981). General principles of psychoanalytic supervision. In *Becoming a Psychoanalyst: A Study of Psychoanalytic Supervision*, ed. R. S. Wallerstein, pp. 29–38. New York: International Universities Press.

Sigman, M. (1985). The parallel process phenomenon in the

supervisory relationship—a therapist's view. *Current Issues in Psychoanalytic Practice* 2:21–31.

Slakter, E. (1987). *Countertransference*. Northvale, NJ: Jason Aronson.

Strean, H. (1984). The patient who would not tell his name. *Psychoanalytic Quarterly* 53:410–420.

——— (1988). *Behind the Couch: Revelations of a Psychoanalyst*. New York: Wiley.

Sullivan, H. S. (1953). *The Interpersonal Theory of Psychiatry*. New York: Norton.

Teitelbaum, S. (1990). Supertransference: the role of the supervisor's blind spots. *Psychoanalytic Psychology* 7(2): 243–258.

Discussion:
The Countertransference
Controversy

Jerrold Brandell

Perhaps no topic in clinical or theoretical psychoanalysis has stimulated greater controversy or been defined in such radically different ways as that of countertransference. As Dr. Strean observes, the earliest references to countertransference viewed it as an obstacle or hindrance to effective psychoanalysis, interfering with the psychoanalyst's full participation in the analytic process, and compromising her analytic neutrality. Countertransference, according to the classical position, represents a psychological "defect" of the analyst that holds "back from consciousness what has been perceived by [the] unconscious" and is therefore, a "blind spot" in the analyst's perception of the patient (Freud 1912, p. 116).

The classical position is anchored in an epistemology of positivism or objectivism, and reflects a view of the clinical process as scientifically determined and knowable. It has been argued that this conception of countertransference adheres to what is termed a *correspondence theory of truth*, a perspective that asserts that all of the critical dimensions of the patient's subjective experience can be systematically scrutinized, if not measured, by the analyst-observer (Hanna

1993, 1998, Mitchell 1993). Within such an epistemology, countertransference attitudes, fantasies, and enactments, in particular, are a serious threat if not a toxic contaminant to the unfolding therapeutic process. They must be understood, but solely for the purpose of eliminating them from the analytic equation lest they impair the analyst's capacity to function as a dispassionate scientist.

As Dr. Strean notes, the classical perspective seems gradually to have been replaced by a far more totalistic conception of countertransference, a development that may suggest that countertransference has achieved a certain level of respectability and acceptance in the psychoanalytic literature. The reasons for this shift in perspective may, however, be somewhat more difficult to identify. The application to social phenomena of Heisenberg's uncertainty principle, originally developed within the framework of the experimental sciences to account for the influence of the observer over his observations, may be one contributing factor. The influence of postmodernism on the behavioral sciences, with its emphasis on the creation of meaning within social and interpersonal contexts, is very likely another major influence. A coterminous development within psychoanalysis, which, as I have suggested elsewhere (Brandell 2000), may be traceable to contributions of the late French psychoanalyst and hermeneuticist Jacques Lacan, is the notion of *intersubjectivity*.

Nearly fifty years ago, Lacan described psychoanalysis as a kind of intersubjective dialogue occurring between subjects, that "retains a dimension which is irreducible to any psychology considered as an objectification of certain properties of the individual" (Lacan 1998, p. xi).[1] Intersubjectivity is now

---

1. Though Lacan does not typically receive credit for his early contributions to the idea of intersubjectivity, this may be due less to poor scholarship on the part of psychoanalytic historians than to the almost mystical quality of his writing, which at times, appears to invite misunderstanding.

most often used to refer to the idea of reciprocal mutual influence in the analytic relationship, or, more narrowly, the continuous interplay between the patient's transference and the analyst's countertransference. This perspective, a natural outgrowth of the shift from a one-person to a two-person psychology, appears to be a radical departure from traditional psychoanalytic ideas about the analytic process and the nature of healing. Thus, some have characterized transference and countertransference, rather than as separate entities arising in response to one another, as being instead "aspects of a single intersubjective totality experienced separately (and individually) by analyst and analysand" (Ogden 1997, p. 25, n. 1). Adherents of an encompassing framework of intersubjectivism have gone even further, describing the intersubjective field as "an indissoluble system that constitutes the empirical domain of psychoanalytic inquiry" (Atwood and Stolorow 1984, p. 64). Within this framework, the effects of the analyst's countertransference on the patient's transference would appear to be no less significant or influential than the effects the patient's transference might exert on the therapist's countertransference. But how do such ideas apply, more specifically, to Dr. Strean's notion of "colluding illusions" in the supervisory situation?

A few words about the history of psychoanalytic supervision may be helpful. In the early days of the psychoanalytic movement, neither supervision nor other aspects of training were formalized; the teaching and supervision of psychoanalytic theory and technique were essentially accomplished through personal apprenticeship. As interest in psychoanalytic training grew in the twenties and thirties, training became more systematic, and by the late thirties, consisted of three basic components: didactic coursework, training analysis, and control analysis (undertaken by the candidate under psychoanalytic supervision). Though there had been strenuous debate as to the advisability of requiring psychoanalytic candidates to be supervised by an analyst other than their

training (personal) analyst, this model prevailed in all institutes except the Hungarian, where the training analyst continued to provide clinical supervision. The Hungarians, under
the leadership of Otto Rank and Sandor Ferenczi, had pro-
moted the idea that the training analyst should also be
responsible for conducting the control analysis. In their view,
this would permit the therapist in training to use "his own
treatment to explore his relationship with his patient and thus
obtain a deeper understanding of his own resistances and
difficulties in conducting analytic work" (Jacobs et al. 1995,
p. 20). The advantages of the Hungarian approach—that the
supervisor had access to the "supervisor's inner life and
deeper understanding of his countertransferences"—were
counterbalanced by the erosion of the "supervisee's sense of
privacy and protection from . . . potentially transference-
laden and intrusive elements of supervision" (p. 24). The
separation of analytic and supervisory functions fostered the
development of a more interactive and collaborative educational dialogue, although it also increased the difficulty of the
supervisory task, requiring the development of a different
model for interaction than that customarily used by the
supervisor with patients.

In effect, the abandonment of the apprenticeship model
and the concomitant separation of the function of training
analysis from that of analytic supervision, has had the effect
of establishing the supervisory encounter as a fundamentally
pedagogic one.[2] Though this model is in many respects
superior to its predecessor, one important consequence of this
bifurcation has been the ambivalence with which many
analytic supervisors undertake exploration of the candidate's

---

2. It should, however, be acknowledged that some consensus
existed as early as 1935 regarding the legitimacy of exploring candidates' countertransference reactions to their patients in the supervisory
encounter (Jacobs et al. 1995), although there has always been considerable variability in the nature and extent of such supervisory dialogues.

countertransference issues, preferring at times to defer such discussions to the candidate's training or personal analyst. In one recent collection of Joan Fleming's papers on psychoanalytic education and supervision, the editor (Weiss) describes the prevailing view of supervision in the following way:

> The predominant view today . . . holds that the supervisor should rely on confronting the student with the presence of a blind spot or defensive reaction to his patient, rather than making transference or genetic interpretations in noting the student's countertransference problems; *the management of such problems should be left to further training analysis or to self-analysis.* [Weiss 1987, pp. xvii–xviii, italics added]

Inasmuch as many analytic supervisors continue to operate under this constraint, the establishment and promotion of a climate wherein the supervising analyst's "supertransference" reactions are likely to be identified and understood, or meaningfully explored (with analyst peers) is probably not a strong likelihood. Stated somewhat differently, the one-person psychology of classical psychoanalytic theory and its counterpart, *objectivism*, continue to serve as a natural philosophical undergirding for the supervisory encounter as it is currently conceived. Such a milieu tends to be infelicitous to *perspectivalism*, a viewpoint that asserts the importance of the personal psychic realities of therapist, patient, and, in this instance, supervisor, and of their reciprocal, mutual influence.

In Dr. Strean's article, the exploration of the supervisor's unconscious collusions with the supervisee and the patient is accomplished through the vehicle of a workshop on psychoanalytic supervision. Although this unusual workshop appears to have been formed as an advanced seminar for supervisors—presumably combining didactic and peer consultation elements—Strean and his colleagues gradually identified the supervisor as having a role in unconsciously promoting certain supervisee–patient collusions and the treatment impasses to which they gave rise. Such a group process is rather exceptional, and obviously required a high degree of professionalism and courage on the part of its participants. In fact, such seminars or workshops for psychoanalytic supervisors may not even be offered at many psychoanalytic institutes.

Nevertheless, the reader is left with the impression that the insights achieved through this unusual group process, to which the supervisee and the patient will be the beneficiaries, are introduced as a fait accompli. The supervisor has sought consultation, identified the therapeutic impasse and his role in unconsciously promoting it, and translocated this new understanding from the workshop milieu back to the supervisory relationship. Because the insight gained by the supervisor occurs with coparticipants in the workshop and *outside of the relationship with the supervisee*, it actually introduces yet another figure into the supervisory equation: that of the *supervisory group's observing ego*. Dr. Strean observes that analytic supervisors and supervisees, like patients, wish to maintain secrets. However, the supervisory model that he proposes, rather than offering a completely satisfactory solution to this problem, may in one sense actually compound it. In each of the case illustrations, the therapeutic/supervisory impasse yields to the supervisor's insights and/or subsequent alterations in supervisory technique, but the process remains a silent one, apparently known only to the supervisor.

Although there is relatively little elaboration on the nature or method of psychoanalytic supervision in each of Dr. Strean's case vignettes, I will make the assumption that these supervisory relationships conformed to the prevailing model of psychoanalytic supervision. As I have suggested above, this model, though useful in many respects, has tended to emphasize educational elements in the supervisory process, focusing less on reciprocal mutual influences of supervisor and supervisee. In one of the most widely referenced texts on psychoanalytic supervision, the supervisor is characterized as "predominantly an educator who follows general educational principles in trying to impart to the candidate various aspects of the analyst's role that must be mastered" (Dewald 1987, p. 9). Dewald then identifies a number of salient supervisory tasks that are presented as a sine qua non for an effective supervisory process. They can be summarized as follows:

1. cognitive didactic instruction
2. demonstration of the thinking process of an analyst
3. listening to clinical material and illustrating the process of clinical inference
4. advising an inexperienced therapist about various technical options
5. encouraging active participation and observation in the student
6. providing prompt and unambiguous feedback regarding progress in learning
7. demonstrating sensitivity to the various affective nuances involved both in the patient's material and in the candidate's presentation during supervision.

Though useful for its time, this model is no longer consonant with contemporary psychoanalytic perspectives emphasizing "the value of not knowing and the courage it requires" (Mitchell 1993, p. 42). This latter position, predicated on the idea that knowledge is perspectival, relativistic, subjective, and bound by social and interpersonal contexts, has exerted a powerful influence on the conduct of psychoanalytic treatment. However, the same influence may not yet have been felt in the manner in which we approach psychoanalytic supervision.

One of the most recent efforts to create a supervisory model sensitive to the sea change that has occurred more

generally in the psychoanalytic approach to knowledge emphasizes the intersubjective basis of the supervisory encounter.
"The supervisory encounter, like the therapeutic encounter, is
coming to be seen as an intersubjective meeting in which each
participant attempts to 'use' the other's subjectivity in order
to grow and develop," a perspective that "changes not only the
balance of power between supervisor and supervisee, but also
the emphases and patterns of relating to interactions within
supervision" (Yerushalmi 1999, pp. 433–434). Yerushalmi
sees several distinct advantages in creating such a basis for
the supervisory process. It may, in the first place, relieve
supervisors of the exclusive responsibility for the growth and
development of their supervisees, inasmuch as such tasks
would instead be seen as mutual and shared. A related point
is that the supervisory discourse is reframed as an opportunity for mutual growth and evolution, rather than solely
focused on the supervisee's professional development. Although didactic learning would continue to be an important
part of the supervisory process, the way in which such
knowledge is both imparted and used will likely differ from
more traditional supervisory encounters. Finally, the nature
of supervisory interaction would become less formalized and
assume greater complexity.

Returning to Dr. Strean's paper, I believe that the development of a supervisory model that emphasizes and values
the subjective experience of both participants and the intersubjective basis of their encounter, and that contextualizes the
transmission of didactic information within such an epistemological framework, may result in several additional salu-
tary effects:

1. It may lessen the likelihood or diminish the potency of
   certain illusory beliefs or heightened transference-like
   expectations of the supervisor (e.g., unconscious beliefs regarding the supervisor's omniscience, illusions

that the supervisor is exempt from pathology, ignorance, or blind spots, or other feelings based on the
power gradient in traditional supervisory relationships).

2. In consequence, the supervisor may feel somewhat
   more freedom to identify and explore the manifestations of his subjective reactions to the material presented *within the context of the supervision itself*,
   without the need for outside consultation.

3. Should such mutual exploration occur within the
   supervisory encounter, it would (a) provide both participants an opportunity to discuss countertransference in a three-dimensional context, and (b) obviate
   the need for the creation of a "silent" third party (*the
   supervisory group's observing ego*) that, while undoubt-
   edly contributing to the supervisor's insights, also
   interferes with the creative potential of an intersubjective supervisory process.

In the foregoing, I have discussed some of the significant
theoretical, epistemological, and pedagogical issues raised by
Dr. Strean's provocative article on colluding illusions. I am in
basic agreement with his position on countertransference,
and, likewise, have no quarrel with his contention that the
supervisor's contribution to a therapeutic impasse between
supervisee and patient may be both powerful and largely
unconscious. My position, however, is two-fold: (1) that such
influences may be somewhat mitigated by a more intersubjective approach to supervision, and (2) when they do occur, it
may prove useful to identify and explore them actively within
the supervisory milieu itself, thereby furthering the candidate's and the supervisor's awareness of the complexity of
dynamic interactive processes and of the counterresistances
and countertransferences each brings to the supervisory encounter.

REFERENCES

Atwood, G., and Stolorow, R. (1984). *Structures of Subjectivity: Explorations in Psychoanalytic Phenomenology*. Hillsdale, NJ: Analytic Press.

Brandell, J. (2000). Listening at the movies. *Readings* 15(1): 6–11.

Dewald, P. (1987). *Learning Process in Psychoanalytic Supervision: Complexities and Challenges*. Madison, CT: International Universities Press.

Freud, S. (1912). Recommendations to physicians practising psychoanalysis. *Standard Edition* 12:111–120.

Hanna, E. (1993). The implications of shifting perspectives on countertransference for the therapeutic action of clinical social work: Part 2: The recent totalist and intersubjectivist positions. *Journal of Analytic Social Work* 1:(3):53–79.

——— (1998). The role of the therapist's subjectivity: using countertransference in psychotherapy. *Journal of Analytic Social Work* 5:(4):1–24.

Jacobs, D., David, P., and Meyer, D. (1995). *The Supervisory Encounter: A Guide for Teachers of Psychodynamic Psychotherapy and Psychoanalysis*. New Haven, CT: Yale University Press.

Lacan, J. (1988). *The Language of the Self*. Baltimore, MD: Johns Hopkins University Press.

Mitchell, S. (1993). *Hope and Dread in Psychoanalysis*. New York: Basic Books.

Ogden, T. (1997). *Reverie and Interpretation: Sensing Something Human*. Northvale, NJ: Jason Aronson.

Weiss, S. (1987). *The Teaching and Learning of Psychoanalysis: Selected Papers of Joan Fleming, M.D.* New York: Guilford.

Yerushalmi, H. (1999). Mutual influences in supervision. *Contemporary Psychoanalysis* 35(3):415–436.

Discussion:
The Unpredictable
Currents of Supervision

Stanley Teitelbaum

We have come a long way in psychoanalytic supervision from the era in which it was perceived primarily in terms of an advanced analyst imparting knowledge to a less experienced analyst or an analytic candidate in training. In this model the supervisor was viewed as the expert who was helpful in deepening an understanding of the patient's material and in exploring and addressing the analyst's unresolved conflicts and overreactions to the patient that reflected countertransference impediments in the treatment situation. When conflicts occurred within the supervisory relationship, it was invariably viewed as emanating from the side of the supervisee, who was struggling with anxiety overexposure, evaluation, problems in learning, and the like. The impact of the supervisory style or the supervisory atmosphere created by the supervisor was seldom addressed as a factor in the difficulties that emerged. It was assumed that the more experienced and well-analyzed supervisor was less likely to be the source of supervisory tensions than the less experienced and less well-analyzed supervisee. We now recognize that in many instances this is a grand illusion, and that the supervisor, while more experienced, brings along her own blind spots that encroach upon the supervisory encounter. Thus, the supervisor may have inappropriate or countertransferential reactions to such things as the supervisee's feelings and attitudes toward the patient, the supervisee's personality, his manner of presenting case material, and so forth. I have referred to these reactions as *supertransference* (Teitelbaum 1990).

Contemporary conceptualization of the supervisory process extends beyond the earlier patient-centered approach and attends to additional dimensions, particularly the ways in which supervisor and supervisee exert a mutual influence upon one another. In this framework such things as invitations to collusion between supervisee and supervisor (along with collusions between patient and supervisee) are recognized, explored, and addressed insofar as they impact on the supervisory and treatment relationships.

In this regard Dr. Strean's article provides a substantial and well–thought-out contribution to contemporary views on psychoanalytic supervision. His article emerged from his collaboration with colleagues in an ongoing psychoanalytic supervision seminar, and it is commendable that Dr. Strean and other senior supervisors created the opportunity to explore important issues in supervision, including their own participation in the treatment impasses of their supervisees. As a result of exchanges like those referred to in Dr. Strean's group, supervisors can become more aware and accepting of their own imperfections, inappropriate expectations, role responsiveness, and tendencies toward collusion. In this way supervisors can productively shift their emphasis away from tensely striving to be experts with super-vision, to a wider scope of variables that affect the treatment process under study.

I believe that supervisory impasses occur much more frequently than has been previously acknowledged, and that we must examine more closely the contributions of the supervisor to these impasses. Dr. Strean astutely calls our attention to this issue in pointing out that "if all psychoanalysts experience and reexperience conflicts in their work, one place where the senior analyst [i.e., the supervisor] will be very prone to countertransference problems is in the supervisory situation." He highlights the importance of the supervisor's openness to looking into the influence of her own current life circumstances (e.g., children leaving the nest, yearning to be a parent again, and so on) and its effect on how one deals with supervisees. He perceptively states that "many supervisors may unconsciously want to use the analytic candidate in the service of buttressing lowered self-esteem, refueling lost narcissism, or finding a lost child." It is noteworthy that to examine the causes of impasse under this type of lens was challenging to the supervisory zeitgeist that existed at the time Dr. Strean's article appeared in 1991 and that was tilted in the direction of attributing impasses to the problems of the "difficult supervisee." In this way Dr. Strean's work is in the forefront of the changing supervisory atmosphere that in many circles has become increasingly egalitarian and collaborative. We can now more readily acknowledge what has always existed, which is that the supervisor, as well as the analyst, brings a set of needs to the supervisory relationship. The supervisor–supervisee relationship is made more complex by these needs, which include the supervisor's legitimate narcissistic needs, such as the wish to mentor, and her more neurotic needs, such as disciple hunting, or competitiveness with the supervisee.

When considering the host of variables that enter into the supervisory alliance (such as divergent expectations, mutual anxieties, legitimate narcissistic needs, the pull toward collusions), it is understandable that some degree of conflict in supervision is more or less inevitable. Misalliances and impasses that are not addressed and remain unresolved frequently lead to a premature termination of the supervision. In a recent study on termination in psychotherapy Hunsley and colleagues (1999) found significantly divergent perspectives between therapists and patients in describing the reasons for termination. Their findings indicated that therapists significantly underestimated the role of dissatisfaction with treatment and the therapist as a central factor in patients' decision to terminate. These authors maintain that therapists tend to have limited awareness of the real reasons governing their patients' decision to end treatment. I believe that a similar discrepancy exists among supervisors and supervisees in understanding the reasons for premature termination in supervision. It therefore behooves the psychoanalytic supervisor to examine her own supertransference issues in the context of an impasse in the supervision and/or in the case under study, in order to attenuate ineffective supervision.

Dr. Strean extends our knowledge of the intricacies of the parallel process phenomenon. It is also worth noting that parallel process refers not only to reenactments from therapy into supervision, but may also occur in the reverse direction (Doehrman 1976). For example a supervisee who is excessively supportive and nonconfrontational with a patient may be reenacting in the treatment the way the supervisor approaches the supervisee. In a seminal paper on supervision Epstein (1986) draws upon Sullivan's concept of selective inattention to highlight the ways in which collusions may develop between supervisor and supervisee to ignore aspects of the supervisor's negative impact on the supervisee. Epstein points out that

> it is striking that the actual emotional impact of the supervisor's conduct of the supervision on the supervisee and on its carry over to the supervisee's conduct of the treatment has received scant attention in the psychoanalytic literature . . . and . . . should the supervisor have an actual aversion to discovering any negative impact he might be having, the

supervisee is likely to join him in a tacit collusion to
be selectively inattentive to such matters. [pp. 390–
391]

In a parallel way the supervisee in this situation may
invite the patient to selectively inattend to her negative
reactions toward the therapist, and a detrimental collusion is
thereby established. Epstein advocates a supervisory approach that encourages the supervisee to express his negative
reactions about the supervisor, the supervision, and the patient, in order to counteract collusions that serve to tone down
the affective components of the supervision, as well as the
patient's treatment.

Case 1 in Dr. Strean's article illustrates how the "mutual
admiration" collusion between supervisor and supervisee
trickled down into the treatment situation, insofar as the
therapist proceeded for quite a while in a way that did not
facilitate the emergence of the patient's hostile fantasies
toward him. As long as the supervisor and supervisee remained locked into what I would call their "no-heat collusion," the teaching and learning about such dimensions as
resistance, negative transference, defenses, and technical interventions were not being sufficiently addressed, with the
result that the patient did not sustain genuine progress. In
this situation the supervisory seminar was invaluable to the
supervisor in opening up his awareness of an interfering
collusion. As we increasingly recognize the complexities involved in psychoanalytic supervision and the propensity for
collusions, the supervisory seminar described here, or what I
would refer to as supervision of the supervision, is an excellent avenue for the supervisor to acquire professional feedback about his or her work with a supervisee.

Case 2 exemplifies the enmeshments in treatment and
supervision that can occur when all three participants have
overlapping unresolved conflicts. In this vignette a break-

through in the supervision occurred when the supervisor recognized that a parallel process had emerged in which the analyst was distancing herself from her supervisor similarly to the way the patient was distancing himself from the analyst. By drawing attention to an impasse in the supervision, and identifying the theme of symbiotic yearnings and defenses mobilized against such longings in himself and in the patient, the supervisor helped the supervisee to better understand and work with these issues in her patient. It was paramount for the supervisor to recognize and address the collusion of avoidance in response to not feeling understood (the patient), and feeling criticized (the supervisee), in order to overcome the ensuing stalemate in the treatment and supervision respectively. It is important to note that when the supervisor recognized that his too proper and too stiff manner was replicating a negative dimension from the treatment situation, he became free to work with this without spelling it out with the supervisee as a parallel process. Many supervisors become fascinated with the concept of parallel process, and they sometimes are too hasty in pointing this out to the supervisee, a tactic that may serve to make the supervisee increasingly defensive. A more selectively judicious approach in the introduction of this phenomenon to the supervisee was recommended by Searles (1955) in his pivotal paper on parallel process. A tactful inquiry is required on the part of the supervisor in approaching the analyst's countertransference issues that may be generated by the pressures of parallel process. Such questions as, "Perhaps we can figure out together what's happening between us—then maybe it will be easier to see what's going on in the treatment?", utilized by the supervisor in Case 2, are especially sensitive in unraveling collusive selective inattention.

In their resolution of the problem between supervisor and analyst and correspondingly between analyst and patient, there may be another collusion operating that was not fully addressed in this vignette. I am referring here to the tendency to understand a treatment impasse exclusively in terms of the patient's dynamics and pathology, which thereby avoids a fuller examination of the validity of the patient's negative reactions toward the analyst. It is shortsighted to believe that negative transference reactions are always solely precipitated by the patient's pathology. In intersubjective terms we need to consider the dimension of mutual influence between patient and analyst in order to fully appreciate the transference–countertransference configurations. From this perspective we need to examine whether Mr. B.'s negativistic reactions to Dr. V. were not only expressions designed to defend himself against wishes to merge, but were also based on his accurate perception of her superanalytic aloofness. It seems possible that Dr. V., as an analytic candidate, was interacting with Mr. B. as a caricature of how a psychoanalyst functions. In other words, perhaps Dr. V.'s analytic demeanor was appropriately experienced as cold, detached, and emotionally unavailable. This is somewhat stylistically typical among beginning analytic candidates who may assume a wooden and mechanical analytic posture as they struggle to find their path toward a comfortable way of working. Thus, by focusing on the patient's conflict around his wishes to merge as an explanation for his negative and distancing reactions to the analyst, the supervisor and analyst may be colluding to avoid looking into the possible legitimate and iatrogenic aspects of the patient's dissatisfaction with Dr. V.

In Case 3 we see again the "collusive selective inattention" described by Epstein (1986) to some deeper meaning of what is going on between the patient–analyst, and analyst–supervisor dyads. Superficial blandness concealed unexpressed angry reactions about disappointments in the treatment and in the supervision. It is easier and less anxiety arousing to view the patient's planned termination entirely as a function of her job offer, rather than to consider to what extent Ms. C.

was using the reality of the job offer in the service of distancing herself from Dr. W.; and that Ms. C. and Dr. W. were colluding to avoid exploring the issues between them that contributed to Ms. C.'s limited progress. Likewise, the supervisor's protective feelings toward the patient and his hostile feelings toward the supervisee were underacknowledged, and contributed to the collusive atmosphere. It is not clear in this vignette how the supervisor dealt with the analyst around the issue of her not being overly distressed about Ms. C. leaving treatment. In addition to the negative connection to his daughter-in-law, was the supervisor's hostility based on his critical feelings toward Dr. W. because she hadn't helped the patient sufficiently? Was he colluding in avoiding exploration of this because of his own concerns about not being of greater help to the supervisee and thereby protecting himself from the emergence of Dr. W.'s rage toward him? These are some of the possible supertransference issues that a supervisor needs to consider in order to be maximally effective. Through an ongoing awareness and examination of supertransference the supervisor will often discover a more productive way to proceed with the supervisee and this will often filter down in a positive way to the analyst–patient relationship. As Dr. Strean aptly surmises in his concluding statement, "If the supervisor becomes aware of his or her role in the collusion, the treatment situation seems to improve markedly for both the analytic candidate and the patient."

Dr. Strean stresses the point that the theoretical perspective of the supervisor will influence the direction of themes that are highlighted in the supervisory exchange. Accordingly, as a classical Freudian, Dr. Strean presents examples in his article that emphasize the role of aggression and sex, and defenses against the expression of these feelings. Supervisors who espouse alternative theoretical orientations would be prone to organize the material in terms of such concepts as selfobject needs, the fear of retraumatization, idealization and devaluation, positive and negative self and object representations, and so forth. The supervisor's theoretical perspective may also influence the extent to which supervision is approached, primarily from a patient-centered, analyst-centered, or supervisory relationship-centered vantage point. The literature has described supervisors with a classical orientation who tend to proceed primarily in a didactic mode, while those who espouse a two-person psychology theoretical framework tend to utilize a more experimental approach (Rock 1997, Teitelbaum 1998). Nevertheless, regardless of theoretical orientation, supervisors need to be ever alert to the propensity for collusion to permeate the treatment and supervisory arenas, and to be able to shift gears and work toward eliminating these impediments. By highlighting the ways in which the supervisor's conflicts can contribute to treatment and supervisory impasses, and by presenting rich case examples, Dr. Strean has provided us with a valuable compass to navigate the unpredictable currents of supervision.

REFERENCES

Doehrman, M. J. (1976). Parallel processes in supervision and psychotherapy. *Bulletin of the Menninger Clinic* 40:9–84.

Epstein, L. (1986). Collusive selective inattention to the negative impact of the supervisory interaction. *Contemporary Psychoanalysis* 22:389–409.

Hunsley, J., Aubry, T., Verstervelt, C., and Veto, D. (1999). Comparing therapist and client perspectives on reasons for psychotherapy termination. *Psychotherapy: Theory, Research, Practice, Training* 36(4):380–388.

Rock, M. (1997). Effective supervision. In *Psychodynamic Supervision*, ed. M. Rock, pp. 107–132. Northvale, NJ: Jason Aronson.

Searles, H. F. (1955). The informational value of the supervisor's emotional experiences. In *Collected Papers on*

Schizophrenia and Related Subjects, pp. 157–176. New York: International Universities Press, 1965.

Teitelbaum, S. (1990). Supertransference: the role of the supervisor's blind spots. *Psychoanalytic Psychology* 7(2): 243–258.

——— (1995). The changing scene in psychoanalytic supervision. *Psychoanalysis and Psychotherapy* 12(2):183–192.

4

Resolving Some Therapeutic Impasses by Disclosing Countertransference

As the previous chapters and their discussions suggest, countertransference is ubiquitous and no clinician is exempt from it. As Jacobs (1986) has argued, psychotherapy is far more related to the personality of the therapist than it is to the therapist's technique. Jacobs views extensive countertransference participation and enactment as inevitable. He refers to subtle metacommunications, usually nonverbal in nature, between patient and therapist as having considerable influence on both parties.

McLaughlin (1981) has suggested that the term *countertransference* should be changed to "the therapist's transference." He views both patient and therapist as primitive and infantile in their participation and believes the patient is as likely to influence the therapist as the reverse. He suggests that countertransference is *always* present in the practitioner and that psychotherapeutic interaction is an engagement between two subjectivities.

Bird (1972) and Sandler (1976) have contended that not only are countertransference responses inevitable but they are *necessary* for the therapist to experience; otherwise, the interaction between patient and therapist will not be fully understood by either of them. In effect, they say that countertransference participation may be an essential ingredient for the patient's reenactment of the transference and therefore is a necessary part of the therapy.

Several writers have been able to document the fact that the clinician's theoretical predilections are very much a function of his unique personality (Cooper 1998, Hirsch 1998, Schafer 1983, Spence 1982, Strean 1975, 1995). As Hirsch (1998) has pointed out, the history of psychotherapy has been "plagued by the divergence of and often disrespect for rival schools of thought" (p. 79). Each perspective has suffered from a failure to integrate what is valuable in other points of view.

Although we clinicians tend to hold onto our theoretical perspectives and therapeutic biases with a certain degree of tenacity, there is no doubt that more of us are moving toward a model of the therapist as a participant-observer. As participant-observers we are tending to accept as given "that when at work [the therapist] *always* processes and thus necessarily modifies that which is being explored by the patient" (Poland 1986, p. 268). Because many more practitioners of different theoretical persuasions are rejecting the classical model of a one-person psychology and viewing therapy more and more as a two-person psychology, with transference and countertransference in constant interaction, the notion of the therapist disclosing his countertransference responses to the patient is becoming accepted by more practitioners. Many therapists believe that because their countertransference reactions influence their patients' productions patients are better helped to understand themselves in more depth and breadth when they become more aware of the social context and interactional field in which the therapy is taking place.

THE EVOLUTION OF DISCLOSING COUNTERTRANSFERENCE REACTIONS AS A THERAPEUTIC PROCEDURE

The Lessening of Authoritarianism

One of the most dramatic changes that has occurred in our society during the last two to three decades is that we have become much more of an egalitarian culture. Class and caste struggles are breaking down, there is increased racial and religious tolerance, men and women understand and respect each other more, and parent–child relationships are moving toward more mutuality. This shift toward more equality in interpersonal relationships has been very much in evidence in the interaction between patient and therapist (Fine 1982).

No longer is the therapeutic dyad conceived of as composed of a wise practitioner and a naive patient (Racker 1968). Instead the therapeutic situation is more frequently viewed as consisting of two vulnerable individuals, "more human than otherwise" (Sullivan 1953), working together to discover the emotional truth that exists between them. In effect, the therapist's role has become much less authoritarian (Maroda 1994).

Balint (1968) has pointed out that when the clinician's technique and behavior are suggestive of omniscience and omnipotence, the greater is the possibility that the patient will feel like a very imperfect child next to a very perfect parent. Inasmuch as more practitioners have been struggling to reduce their authoritarian stance in the therapeutic situation, they have begun to question the helpfulness of professional distance, therapeutic abstinence, and therapeutic anonymity.

It has been suggested that therapeutic procedures such as not answering patients' questions, intervening exclusively through interpretation, and showing limited emotion in the therapeutic situation may actually distort and inhibit the transference that could have developed in a more reciprocal relationship (Maroda 1994).

As clinicians have noted the negative effects of a strict environment in child rearing and elsewhere, they have recognized that a strict and rigid authoritarian atmosphere in the therapy can stifle and inhibit the patient from freely showing transference reactions and other affects. Many patients who feel compelled to obey the fundamental rule tend to repress their hostility and idealize the therapist, but in a nonproductive manner. In effect, the traditional authoritarian atmosphere that often promotes reaction formations and unspontaneous patient behavior in sessions has yielded to a more reciprocal relationship between patient and therapist. As the therapist is freer to show his affects, vulnerabilities, and anxieties, particularly as they are felt countertransferentially, patients have become freer to express a wider range of emotion in the therapy, particularly as they experience their affects in the transference (Strean 1993).

During the past couple of decades, with role reciprocity between patient and therapist considered more a fact of therapeutic life, the patient has emerged as an untapped source of strength who can instruct the therapist and keep the latter on track (Schafer 1983). It is now recognized that the patient can not only serve as a consultant to the therapist (Strean 1998), but can actually be less conflicted about certain issues than the therapist is. Consequently, therapists, after acknowledging certain hangups of their own, may, with the patient's understanding and empathy, become empowered to function as more empathetic and secure practitioners.

The nonauthoritarian atmosphere that has been permeating much of our work has encouraged practitioners to feel more freely their patients' feelings. The popularity of Kohut

(1977) may be attributed in part to his encouraging therapists to feel what their patients feel. In the past, this was often taboo and served to maintain a big distance between therapist and patient. Kohut's permission for therapists to be as human and vulnerable as they try to help their patients become has been liberating to many clinicians.

As the distance between therapists and patients is diminishing, therapists are less phobic and less paranoid in the therapeutic situation. Patients are not as frequently experienced as adversaries out to derail treatment. Thus, as is true in any human relationship, when the partners feel less threatened by each other, they are more inclined to share their feelings. This can include statements by the therapist such as, "Yes, you've gotten to me and I'm upset by your constant criticism [or anything else that hurts or upsets the practitioner]. I'd like to understand better what's happening between us that is arousing feelings in me and that is interfering with our work."

The Therapist Becomes More of a Human Being

Michael Sussman (1992) studied the unconscious motivations of those individuals who choose psychotherapy as a career. In his very thorough empirical study, Sussman was able to document that the modal therapist is a "wounded healer." Frequently suffering from many neurotic conflicts, trying to cope with a present that seems like a tortured past, the wounded healer is psychologically very similar to his patients and often the latter have it more together than their therapeutic counterparts.

As more clinicians have confronted the fact that they bring as many unresolved difficulties to the therapeutic encounter as their patients do, they have been more willing to view the healing process as one in which both parties wish to grow. Searles (1973) has written of the patient's need to heal the "afflicted mother" and has noted that the emergence of this attitude in the treatment is usually indicative of a blossoming transference. He concludes that we as therapists seek to be healed ourselves and we heal our old "afflicted" caretakers as we heal our patients.

During the last two decades, as patients and therapists became "more human than otherwise," the therapeutic community and our consumers have become more realistic about the limitations of psychotherapy and have recognized that it does not provide a complete cure for everybody. This has induced a feeling of humility in most therapists and certainly has helped create an attitude that therapy can be more mutual and reciprocal, with both parties helping to enhance the process. During the last couple of decades therapists have begun to consult their patients in order to break therapeutic stalemates (Maroda 1994, Strean 1998).

In sum, the last twenty years have produced a climate within the psychotherapeutic establishment in which a more mutual relationship between practitioner and patient is advocated. Openness and nondefensiveness on the part of the therapist is championed and therefore the therapist's disclosure of his countertransference is becoming much more acceptable as a therapeutic procedure. As the interpersonal aspects of the therapeutic relationship are more widely recognized and accepted, the anonymity of the practitioner becomes unrealistic.

WHEN TO DISCLOSE THE COUNTERTRANSFERENCE

Although countertransference is viewed by most clinicians as an ever-present fact of therapeutic life, there is considerable disagreement about how it should be utilized in the therapeutic situation. Tansey and Burke (1989) have categorized disclosure practices as conservative, moderate, and radical. Conservatives such as Reich (1960), Heimann (1950), and Langs (1978) take the position that although being aware of countertransference reactions is useful to the therapist, disclosing them is burdensome to the patient and unnecessarily indulgent for the therapist. Moderates such as Giovacchini (1972) and Winnicott (1949) believe that occasional disclosure is appropriate, but only with more seriously disturbed patients. Little (1951), Bollas (1983), Maroda (1994), and Searles (1979) have been termed "radical" because they favor active disclosure of the countertransference and do see it as an integral part of sound treatment.

Despite the fact that there are those who advocate frequent disclosure of the countertransference (for example the Radicals according to Goldstein [1994], Tansey and Burke [1989]), it is difficult to locate any author who has been able to offer clear and specific guiding principles that can help us determine when disclosure of the countertransference is an appropriate therapeutic procedure.

Little (1951) was one of the first to advocate countertransference disclosure. She discussed how the interplay of transference and countertransference led to a mutual regression that threatened the equilibrium of the therapist. Little averred that the only way to avoid being overwhelmed by this experience was to admit one's countertransference to the patient. The therapist must disclose whatever is necessary to facilitate the patient's awareness and acceptance of the truth.

Gitelson (1952) suggested that one "can reveal as much of oneself as is needed to foster and support the patient's discovery of the reality of the actual interpersonal situation as contrasted with the transference–countertransference situation" (p. 7).

Gorkin (1987) reviewed literature on countertransference disclosure and stated the following as the reasons for doing so.

1. to confirm the patient's sense of reality
2. to establish the therapist's honesty or genuineness
3. to establish the therapist's humanness
4. to clarify both the fact and the nature of the patient's impact on the therapist, and on people in general, and
5. to break through a negative therapeutic reaction [pp. 85–86]

Maroda (1994) suggests that what should govern disclosure of the countertransference is the following:

> The therapist must disclose whatever is necessary to facilitate the patient's awareness and acceptance of the truth. And the guiding principle for how and when this is done is simple. The timing, nature, and extent of the countertransference disclosed can only be determined by the therapist in consultation with the patient. [p. 87]

Hirsch (1980–1981) has discussed the inevitability of feelings of envy and resentment in the therapist and points out:

> Our patients are often younger, smarter, in better health, better looking, have more potential, have more excitement in their lives, have better relationships with their loved ones, have more money, and on and on. [Therapists] who are unable to acknowledge both the fact of such differences and the ensuing jealousy or competitiveness run the risk of acting unconsciously to stifle the patient. [p. 127]

Different authors have indicated that therapists should learn to relate comfortably to feelings that patients have difficulty expressing, such as sexual and aggressive ones (Kernberg 1975, Maroda 1994, Searles 1975, Winnicott 1949).

Kernberg (1975) has discussed the inevitable feelings of anger, frustration, and hopelessness that are stimulated in therapists who work with borderline personalities. Searles (1975) has noted that, particularly with very regressed patients, the therapist will naturally regress to primitive sexual and aggressive strivings and should acknowledge these feelings to the patient. Maroda (1994) has suggested, "But just as sex and aggression cause the most difficulties for our patients, so do they for us as therapists. It is seldom that one hears any reference to hating a patient or being sexually attracted to a patient that is accepted as natural" (p. 90). Winnicott (1949) has pointed out that we cannot be helpful to our patients when they are feeling hateful or erotic if we cannot accept these feelings in ourselves.

Despite the fact that disclosure of the countertransference is considered a legitimate therapeutic procedure by many and although some guiding principles regarding its use have been considered, there is still a dearth of information as to its timeliness, specificity, and appropriateness. Whether it is helpful to the patient at the very beginning of treatment has been discussed and debated by clinical social workers (Raines and Strean 1997). Cooper (1998) has discussed countertransference disclosure in which the therapist attempts to make explicit to the patient how the therapist experiences something during a session that differs from the way the patient experiences the same moment. Authors such as Hirsch (1980–1981), Langs (1978), and Slakter (1987) have suggested that countertransference disclosure is appropriate only when the therapist has erred and the error has interfered with therapeutic progress.

During the past several years I have found that disclosing my countertransference reactions was most helpful to my patients (and to me) when there was a therapeutic impasse. I am using the dictionary definition of the term: "a position or situation from which there is no logical way out; a deadlock"

(*Winston Dictionary* 1943). I have felt that there was no logical way out on many occasions and some of them are as follows:

1. The patient did not want to face certain affects or conflicts that I felt were crucial to the treatment. The patient fought my suggestions regarding releasing affects and/or facing certain conflicts, and I could not comfortably respect her resistances.
2. The patient did not want to confront certain transference reactions that were obvious to me, and therapy began to appear more like a debate rather than an exploration of transference resistances.
3. I could not comfortably explore with the patient certain characteristics that he saw in me. My deflection of the patient's positive or negative transference reactions interfered with therapeutic progress.
4. The patient and/or I could not confront dependent, sexual, or tender feelings toward each other, and the treatment began to feel dull and boring for at least one of us (and usually for both of us).
5. The patient and I were competing without resolution.
6. The patient's grasp of reality seemed very tenuous to me, and I began to feel very anxious, worried about the patient regressing too much.
7. The patient accepted all of my interventions but did not make any significant progress.
8. The patient rejected all of my interventions, telling me that I was not understanding her and in many ways implied that I did not know what I was doing.

A few qualifications should be mentioned about the above list. First, the eight items are not mutually exclusive. It was quite possible, for example, for the patient and/or me to feel competitive (Number 5) and for the patient to reject all of my interpretations (Number 8) at the same time. Second, all of the items in the above list that induced me eventually to share any current countertransference reactions with the patient were discovered in hindsight. To quote Renik (1993) again, "awareness of countertransference is always retrospective, preceded by a countertransference enactment" (p. 556). Third, the nature of the patient behavior that induced strong countertransference reactions in me may or may not have induced them in another therapist. Hence, if another therapist did not react the way I did to the patient's productions, there would be less likelihood for a therapeutic impasse to have occurred and perhaps even less likelihood for another therapist to disclose countertransference reactions.

The following section presents short vignettes that involved therapeutic impasses for me with specific patients. I will briefly describe the impasse, state the specific content of the self-disclosure, and then describe the patient's reaction to my disclosure of my countertransference. This will be followed by a full discussion of what transpired in all of the cases.

CASE EXAMPLES

A Disavowal of Affect

Many patients who come to us for therapy are very frightened to reveal their affects. Although it may be very clear that these patients are feeling hostile, sad, or depressed, our attempts to help them confront their affects are strongly resisted. This, in turn, can induce strong countertransference reactions in us.

Amy, a 30-year-old woman who had spent several years in a mental hospital, had been abused both sexually and physically very early in her life. At the age of 2 and until she was an adolescent, she was frequently raped by a psychotic grandfather who was often encouraged to do so by her schizophrenic mother (the grandfather's daughter).

In Amy's initial contacts with me, she was full of self-hate, blamed herself continually for her miserable and depressed life, and rejected all of my interventions that were designed to weaken her punitive superego and give her permission to own her own rage. For example, when I would suggest to Amy that she was having difficulty feeling her hurt and anger toward her grandfather and mother, she would respond by telling me that if she had been a decent person she would not have been "beaten" by her grandfather and mother and would have a better job than being a lowly secretary. She also contended that if she were not disgusting, she would have a decent man in her life. When I tried to help her see that she was punishing herself for her strong hostile and erotic fantasies, she avoided me.

As I got to know Amy better, she began to remind me of a little girl who needed a kind of parental figure to show her how upset he was with the way she had been treated (something I occasionally did as a child therapist with abused children). In the fourth month of twice-a-week therapy, I told Amy how angry I was at her grandfather for raping her and how much I wanted to scream at her mother for condoning this. In response to this disclosure of mine, Amy said, "You're different from all the other shrinks I've had. You really care!" For a couple of months after this intervention she was on a high. She took a job in the theater department of a large university and started to date men who were not as abusive as their predecessors.

After a prolonged therapy honeymoon of two months, Amy then became very paranoid with me and told me I really didn't care very much about her or her life. When I tried to show her that she was afraid to trust me or feel intimate toward me, she insisted that I was a phony.

However, when I eventually shared with her how helpless and unappreciated I was feeling in response to her constantly labeling me a phony, she welcomed my authenticity and began to have erotic fantasies toward me.

Amy did not have much difficulty verbalizing her erotic fantasies toward me and this surprised me, given the story of her life. When I asked her how she experienced herself as she discussed having various types of sex with me, Amy told me that she wanted to see if I could be seduced and was glad that I couldn't be. Soon after her talking about her testing me, she told me that she had strong wishes that I be her father. Although shocked when I said I'd love to have a daughter like her, she gradually moved into a very positive therapeutic alliance, fantasying often that she would sit on my lap and I would tell her stories that demonstrated how much I loved her—something that had never occurred during her childhood.

This patient, though formally well-educated, had a history of emotionally impoverished and self-destructive relationships as well as a poor work record. However, after four years of twice-a-week therapy, she is now happily married, about to give birth to a baby, and is a very successful instructor in a leading university. Treatment continues within a positive therapeutic alliance, with Amy doing a great deal of constructive self-examination and analyzing her transference reactions with much creativity and enthusiasm.

A Power Struggle

A therapeutic impasse is often created when therapist and patient feel negated and unappreciated by each other. Usually one or both parties are unaware of how or why they are provoking each other. To resolve the impasse in which therapist and patient constantly feel attacked, I have found that disclosing the current countertransference reaction can be very helpful. The following two cases are attempts to address this issue:

> Bella, a professional woman wrestler, was referred to me because she was in constant fights with everyone with whom she had contact. It was clear to me the day I met Bella that, as a product of a broken family, she used her strong, aggressive demeanor as a defense to ward off feelings of closeness and vulnerability. Bella was taller, broader, and much tougher than I ever was, and I often felt afraid of her.
>
> In the treatment Bella constantly demeaned me, told me I was "a weak fairy," and that I could not help a soul. Interpretations suggesting that she wanted to defeat me, weaken me, scare me, got nowhere. What she did in response to my interventions was to mock me more. When I told Bella that I thought she wanted to get me very angry and put me in a fighting mood, she picked up a chair and told me, "I'm going to beat the shit out of you!" She then asked, "Are you scared?" Quivering, I said spontaneously, "I'm scared shitless. You can beat me up and I think you will." At this, she put down the chair and said, "I'm proud of you, Herby!" and shook my hand.
>
> When Bella observed that I felt relieved that she was not going to beat me up, she told me that she respected me because I was honest about my fears. Bella also taught me a lesson that I have never forgotten. She stated, "If you had told me earlier in the game that you were furious with me, we could have had a better dialogue." Bella was also able to make another very insightful interpretation. After our struggle subsided, she said, "I got you to express all of the terror that I was unwilling to express. Now I seem freer to be myself with you."

Bella eventually did share with me the hurt and the hate that she had never discussed with a soul. She brought out further that she never felt she was important to anybody and if the court had not insisted that she see me for therapy (because she was involved in theft) she probably never would have tried to get help from anybody. She later said "I think I matter to you."

From a tense relationship in which Bella was very aggressive and I was very intimidated, our therapeutic alliance grew by leaps and bounds after my self-disclosure. Bella completed her therapy several years ago. She is no longer a wrestler; she is a successful social worker and child therapist who still stays in touch with me and calls me "the good doctor."

A transference–countertransference phenomenon that has not been discussed very much in the literature is that colleagues and patients are unconsciously telling us what they are feeling toward us when they refer us patients, and, of course, we are doing the same when we refer patients (Strean 1976).

Several years ago a colleague of mine was winding down his practice to semi-retire. He kept the patients he liked and referred out those toward whom he had less love. I was referred the case of a 31-year-old man, Charlie, who fought continually with his wife, his colleagues at work, his friends, and, of course, with his previous therapist.

In his first interview with me, Charlie brought in a psychotherapy journal and burlesqued the author's ideas and language. He told me his previous therapist had gotten rid of him but had kept other patients. In his second interview he questioned my fee policy, my vacation schedule, and my "unpleasant" waiting room. Everything about me was no good, and as soon as I opened my mouth to utter a word, he engaged in a filibuster. After

about two months of feeling constantly attacked, de-
meaned, and quite irritated, I told Charlie, "You are
pissing me off! Every time I talk and want to work with
you, I feel frustrated by you because the only thing you
want is to fight with me!" After yelling at me for a couple
of minutes and telling me that I was a weak sister who
can't take it, Charlie became quite subdued and said, "I'm
glad I reached you. I thought you'd just shut up like I
always did with my older brother when he twisted my
arm behind my back and wouldn't let go. If you think I
made you suffer, you should have seen how much my
brother made me suffer."

Charlie could then discuss with me how he had been
doing to practically everybody what his brother had done
to him. With this insight, his marriage and work improved a great deal and he became much more willing to
discuss his traumatic past and share his vulnerable
feelings with me. Treatment continues and the therapeutic alliance is quite positive.

Some Dependency Problems

Another type of therapeutic impasse that self-disclosure
seems to help resolve is when the patient has strong resistance
to depending on the therapist for help. The following illustrates how my countertransference disclosure resolved the
impasse.

David, a 46-year-old man, was an Orthodox Jew but also
an atheist. When he came to see me he was indignant
because he could not find a woman who was also an
Orthodox Jewish atheist. Furthermore, David was very
angry at the four therapists he had already seen prior to
meeting me because they failed to help him find a
solution to his problem.

A brilliant scientist with a Ph.D. from a prestigious university, David spent most of his time in his sessions deriding his colleagues at work, the women he met, his parents and family, and me. He was quite critical of anything I said. When I made interpretations regarding his need to keep a distance from me, he rejected them. If I tried to show him that what he was doing with me in the transference paralleled what he did with others— reject them—David told me I was not objective and quite unscientific.

After feeling angry, helpless, and frustrated for several months, I disclosed my countertransference reactions to David. I told him of a fantasy I had and said, "Every time I enter your house you slam the door shut, and I'm forced to be all by myself, feeling thrown out." David retorted, "I let you in but you have nothing valuable to offer. You talk like a rabbi and think you know it all." When I asked David to help me understand my "dogmatism" and "imperiousness" better, he was eventually able to liken me to his Orthodox Jewish mother who always controlled every part of his life, which he hated.

As a result of my self-disclosure, David clarified for me his transference toward me, of which I was completely oblivious. My patient wanted to see me as his authoritarian Orthodox Jewish mother with whom he always fought. My unwillingness to see myself this way (my countertransference) exacerbated David's resistance to work with me, and this in turn intensified my countertransference.

When David and I could discuss how we alienated each other, it strengthened our therapeutic alliance and made for much progress. David now dates women more regularly and is much more relaxed with them. (After relating to the disclosure of my countertransference,

David did manage to find a woman to date who was an Orthodox Jew but also an atheist!) Treatment continues.

A Negative Therapeutic Reaction

The classical negative therapeutic reaction wherein the patient acknowledges, agrees, and repeats all of the therapist's interpretations with seeming insight but makes no therapeutic progress may be helped by the therapist's disclosure of his countertransference. It seems to release the sadism that is usually the prime mover of the negative therapeutic reaction.

> Ellen, a 48-year-old woman with a poor history of relationships with men and an equally poor history with therapists, sought my help because of severe phobias, psychosomatic problems, no sexual pleasure, and depression. Always praising me, always seeing "the truth" in my observations, Ellen made very few gains in therapy.
>
> When I found myself feeling manipulated and irritated by Ellen's ingratiating demeanor for over three months, I shared with her that I felt very depreciated because I thought she never leveled with me. I also told her that I continually felt that I was being "brownnosed." At first full of tears, but later with much rage, Ellen told me how she felt the only way to get along in this world was "to lick ass." My self-disclosure released much of Ellen's sadism, reduced her psychosomatic problems to virtually zero, and brought her much closer to people.

DISCUSSION OF CASES

What can we learn from the vignettes that I have briefly presented?

As we reflect on some of the more prominent dynamics of the patients, we see that they all suffered from poor interpersonal relationships. Either they were very detached from family, friends, and colleagues and/or were very hostile toward them. Loving feelings were not apparent in any of the patients under discussion. If a diagnostic label were to be utilized many of these patients would be called borderline. Considering their impoverished object relations it was understandable that they would find it difficult to relate to the therapists they had seen. Of course, the same phenomenon occurred when they came into treatment with me. Most of the patients could neither trust me nor depend on me as a helper. In several cases they were quite contemptuous of me and the therapy I was trying to provide. Because I genuinely wanted to help these patients but found that my efforts to do so were strongly opposed, I reacted with feelings of hurt, frustration, irritation, alienation, helplessness, boredom, revenge, or with a combination of these feelings. It would appear that my patients and I managed to re-create interactions similar to those they experienced in their daily lives wherein there was much mutual alienation and negative affect.

Inasmuch as traditional interventions designed to resolve therapeutic impasses did not bear much fruit, I decided to disclose my current countertransference reactions to each of these patients. When I did so, we witnessed rather dramatic responses to the affective disclosures. Each patient began to oppose me much less and instead moved toward a more positive therapeutic alliance. As they developed a more trusting relationship with me and could feel safer to express their feelings, particularly feelings of vulnerability, they began to relate to their environments in a more mature fashion. In effect, I believe the disclosure of my countertransference reactions eventually provided a corrective emotional experience for my patients. Why do I say that disclosure of my countertransference reactions helped these five people? Several hypotheses come to mind.

I believe that particularly with the patients under discussion, a one-person psychology with an exclusive focus on their dynamics makes them feel even more vulnerable, more unsafe, more distrusting, and more hostile. These are individuals who either directly or indirectly said that people did not care about them. To share intimate feelings with someone who appears to be uncaring and emotionally unavailable arouses severe anxiety and much paranoia. It does not make for a positive therapeutic alliance.

When the format of the therapy changes to a two-person psychology wherein the patients emotionally perceive that they have an obvious impact on the therapist, their self-esteem rises and they feel less hostile and more friendly toward the practitioner. Observing that the practitioner reacts to them emotionally, and sometimes quite strongly, seems to induce in these patients the feeling that, indeed, they are "a somebody" and as at least four of the patients stated or implied, "You really care."

One of the most obvious features of disclosure of countertransference reactions is that therapists abdicate the role-set of the omnipotent and omniscient parental figure. Sensing that the therapist is not an all-knowing, detached scientist seems to help these patients feel safer in showing their humanness because the therapist is sharing his.

As the patients observed that I was taking some initiative in disclosing my feelings of hurt, anger, rejection, and so forth, they felt a freedom to identify with me and do the same. (And, when I had not revealed very much, they also did the same.) In effect, the therapist was frequently experienced as a role model, as one who set the tone of the interaction. If I was revealing, the patient was more inclined to be revealing. If I withheld, the patient was also withholding.

One of the positive effects of disclosing the current countertransference is that it helps clarify the current transference reaction of the patient. This is particularly helpful when the therapist is unaware of the patient's current transference reaction, as was particularly true in the case of David. But in every case when I told these patients how I was experiencing them, they could tell me with considerable clarity how they were experiencing me.

Most of the patients under discussion induced feelings of being negated, unappreciated, and not cared for in me. When I could share with them that I felt rejected, they were more able to share with me some of the rejection they had felt in their developmental years. This, in turn, lessened their omnipresent defenses and helped them become able to communicate more freely and with a wider range of feelings.

In reviewing the treatment of these patients I became aware that if I had had similar patients in the past, there would have been several premature terminations. I believe that disclosing of the countertransference when there is a therapeutic impasse helps keep the patient in treatment and helps the therapist want to continue working with the patient.

CONCLUSION

Patients who have weak object relations and tend to resist therapy induce strong countertransference responses that alienate them further from the therapist and create a therapeutic impasse. When the therapist shares current countertransference reactions with the patient, the patient's self-esteem rises, and the therapeutic alliance grows stronger. The positive therapeutic alliance becomes replicated in the patient's life with a real growth in the quality and quantity of the patient's object relations.

It is hoped that further research on the therapist's disclosure of the countertransference will be conducted. Is disclosure of the countertransference helpful with other diagnostic groups that were not discussed in this paper? How helpful is self-disclosure when the clinician uses other therapeutic modalities, such as marital counseling or group therapy? Are there other strategic times in therapy in addition to therapeutic impasses when self-disclosure can enhance the patient's psychosocial functioning?

REFERENCES

Abend, S. (1982). Serious illness in the analyst: countertransference considerations. *Journal of the American Psychoanalytic Association* 30:365–379.

Balint, M. (1968). *The Basic Fault*. London: Tavistock.

Bird, B. (1972). Notes on transference: universal phenomenon and hardest part of analysis. *Journal of the American Psychoanalytic Association* 20:267–301.

Bollas, C. (1983). Expressive uses of the countertransference. *Contemporary Psychoanalysis* 19:1–34.

Cooper, S. (1998). Countertransference disclosure and the conceptualization of analytic technique. *Psychoanalytic Quarterly* 67:128–154.

Fine, R. (1982). *The Healing of the Mind*, 2nd ed. New York: Free Press.

Giovacchini, P. (1972). Interpretation and definition of the analytic settings. In *Tactics and Techniques in Psychotherapy*, vol. 1, ed. P. Giovacchini, pp. 291–304. New York: Jason Aronson.

Gitelson, M. (1952). The emotional position of the analyst in the psychoanalytic situation. *International Journal of Psycho-Analysis* 33:1–10.

Goldstein, E. (1994). Self-disclosure in treatment: what the therapists do and don't talk about. *Clinical Social Work Journal* 22:417–433.

Gorkin, M. (1987). *The Uses of Countertransference*. Northvale, NJ: Jason Aronson.

Heimann, P. (1950). On countertransference. *International Journal of Psycho-Analysis* 31:81–84.

Hirsch, I. (1980–1981). Authoritarian aspects of the psychoanalytic relationship. *Review of Existential Psychology and Psychiatry* 17:105–133.

——— (1998). The concept of enactment and theoretical convergence. *Psychoanalytic Quarterly* 67:78–101.

Jacobs, T. (1986). On countertransference enactments. *Journal of the American Psychoanalytic Association* 43:289–307.

Kernberg, O. (1975). *Borderline Conditions and Pathological Narcissism.* New York: Jason Aronson.

Kohut, H. (1977). *The Restoration of the Self.* New York: International Universities Press.

Langs, R. (1978). *The Listening Process.* New York: Jason Aronson.

Little, M. (1951). Countertransference and the patient's response to it. *International Journal of Psycho-Analysis* 32:32–40.

Maroda, K. (1994). *The Power of Countertransference.* Northvale, NJ: Jason Aronson.

McLaughlin, J. (1981). Transference, psychic reality, and countertransference. *Psychoanalytic Quarterly* 50:639–664.

Poland, W. (1986). The psychoanalyst's words. *Psychoanalytic Quarterly* 55:244–272.

Racker, H. (1968). *Transference and Countertransference.* New York: International Universities Press.

Raines, J., and Strean, H. (1997). Dialogue with authors. *Clinical Social Work Journal* 25(3):365–368.

Reich, A. (1960). Further remarks on countertransference. *International Journal of Psycho-Analysis* 32:25–31.

Renik, O. (1993). Analytic interaction: conceptualizing technique in light of the analyst's irreducible subjectivity. *Psychoanalytic Quarterly* 62:553–571.

Sandler, J. (1976). Countertransference and role responsiveness. *International Review of Psycho-Analysis* 3:43–48.

Schafer, R. (1983). *The Analytic Attitude.* New York: Basic Books.

Searles, H. (1973). Concerning therapeutic symbiosis. *Annual of Psychoanalysis* 1:247–262.

—— (1975). The patient as therapist to his analyst. In *Tactics and Techniques in Psychoanalytic Therapy*, vol. 2, ed. P. Giovacchini, pp. 95–151. New York: Jason Aronson.

—— (1979). *Countertransference and Related Studies*. New York: International Universities Press.

Slakter, E. (1987). *Countertransference*. Northvale, NJ: Jason Aronson.

Spence, D. (1982). *Narrative Truth and Historical Truth: Meaning and Interpretation in Psychoanalysis*. New York: Norton.

Strean, H. (1975). *Personality Theory and Social Work Practice*. Metuchen, NJ: Scarecrow Press.

—— (1976). Some psychodynamics in referring a patient for psychotherapy. In *Crucial Issues in Psychotherapy*, ed. H. Strean, pp. 130–139. Metuchen, NJ: Scarecrow Press.

—— (1993). *Resolving Counterresistances in Psychotherapy*. New York: Brunner/Mazel.

—— (1995). Countertransference and theoretical predilections as observed in some psychoanalytic candidates. *Canadian Journal of Psychoanalysis* 3(1):105–123.

—— (1998). *When Nothing Else Works: Innovative Interventions with Intractable Individuals*. Northvale, NJ: Jason Aronson.

Sullivan, H. (1953). *Interpersonal Theory of Psychiatry*. New York: Norton.

Sussman, M. (1992). *A Curious Calling: Unconscious Motivations of Practicing Psychotherapy*. Northvale, NJ: Jason Aronson.

Tansey, M., and Burke, W. (1989). *Understanding Countertransference: From Projective Identification to Empathy*. Hillsdale, NJ: Analytic Press.

Winnicott, D. (1949). Hate in the countertransference. *International Journal of Psycho-Analysis* 30:69–74.

Winston Dictionary (1943). Chicago, IL: John C. Winston.

Discussion:
Flushing Out the Elephants:
My Correspondence with Strean

Barbara Pizer

Although we have never met or spoken in person, Dr. Strean and I have been carrying on a rather refreshing and unusual relationship since 1997. "Dear Dr. Pizer," he wrote, "I have completed reading your very fine article, 'When the Analyst Is Ill: Dimensions of Self-Disclosure,' and I would like to apply for membership in your fan club" (Strean, personal correspondence 1997). Since then, we have been sending our papers to each other and returning critical comments back and forth. It seems to have grown into a two-person mutual admiration society. I hasten to add that our "society" is not founded on automatic agreement. Rather, we share a basic love, awe, and respect for the work we do and the people with whom we do it. We both are interested in issues of countertransference, its use, and its effect in the clinical situation. What I admire most about Herb is that alongside his erudition, his long tenure in our field, he retains the enthusiasm of a schoolboy for the learning and testing out of new ideas. If I were to characterize our differences, I suspect they would not be in the way we ultimately experience and work with our patients. From a stylistic standpoint, Herb has a more systematic, step-by-step method of setting out his clinical arguments while I attempt to convey ideas and meanings via a more evocative approach. Theoretically, Herb puts it this way: "Your criticisms of the paper on sports psychology are valid. As you may have surmised, I've been a classical Freudian analyst for many decades. I have always experimented though, and am still evolving. I think the enclosed talk, which I will put into an article (currently this chapter), puts me in the middle between where I used to be and where you are now" (Strean, personal correspondence 1998). Nevertheless, even though Herb's psychoanalytic roots are perhaps more steeped in a classical tradition while my perspective grows out of the interpersonal and relational "schools," we seem to keep meeting each other in that very middle! So this time, in agreement with the basic ideas in Strean's chapter, I propose to offer a kind of texture to this discussion by bringing something of my own person to it and by starting out from another perspective. And let us see if we do indeed meet in the middle.

As Strean concludes his paper, he writes: "It is hoped that further research on the therapist's disclosure of the counter-transference will be conducted. Is disclosure of the counter-transference helpful with other diagnostic groups that were not discussed in this paper? . . . Are there other strategic times in therapy in addition to therapeutic impasses when self-disclosure can enhance the patient's psychosocial func-tioning?" What if we asked these questions from a different vantage point? Given that most of us believe the therapeutic endeavor involves a two-person relationship, which implies that both parties contribute to the state of health in the dyad, why not begin our research by putting aside the diagnosis we assign to patients? Why not focus our attention on an assess-ment profile, or preliminary inventory, of self-disclosures? As for locating other strategically specific therapy situations where self-disclosure might enhance ongoing process, I think the question places undue limits on what we are looking to understand. Particularly, if we believe with Strean that despite its increased use in the consulting room we still have few definitive guiding principles to help determine when counter-transference disclosure is an appropriate therapeutic proce-dure, why don't we pose the question in reverse? That is to say: When is countertransference disclosure *not* appropriate as a therapeutic procedure in the two-person relationship? In other words, if we accept that the therapeutic endeavor involves two people engaged in focusing on one person's life, we could begin by saying that self-disclosure is therapeuti-cally inappropriate when it derails this ongoing focus. For example, when the therapist defends herself against the deepening affect in the room by relating an amusing associa-tion, the self-disclosure might be considered inappropriate. However, if noticing a change in the therapist's demeanor interrupts the patient's process and he needs to check out his perception, a conspicuous silence on the therapist's part might be equally inappropriate.

So from this point of view, let us consider a preliminary inventory of self-disclosure and when such disclosure is inappropriate. Then we can decide whether in fact we have contributed to Dr. Strean's request for further research.

It was in my article (Pizer 1997)—the one that evoked Strean's fan club application—that I proposed three dimen-sions of analyst disclosure; inescapable, inadvertent, and deliberate. (These dimensions were taken up a year later by David Feinsilver [1998], and I will refer to his work presently.) In a footnote to my paper I wrote:

> Obviously, these aspects of self-disclosure overlap in actual clinical process, and my own particular sys-tem of conceptualizing these component dimen-sions of a total process . . . is arbitrary. But I believe that the mental discipline inherent in utiliz-ing a systematic approach (despite its inevitable shortcomings) serves the function of "checks and balances" on the necessarily intuitive and authentic

responsiveness of the analyst engaged in the current
of a clinical moment. [p. 452]

Inescapable self-disclosure refers to the therapist's acting
on her impression that there is indeed "an elephant in the
room," and that not to mention it would be disconcerting at
best and crazy-making at worst. The precipitating example in
my paper had to do with the intrusive presence of my breast
cancer. This meant an unavoidable surgical schedule just
before vacation that would then be followed, on my return, by
the disruption of chemotherapy every three weeks. I should
add the generalization, however, that while "the elephant in
the room"—emanating from either the patient or from the
therapist's own physical, psychological, or situational state—
feels "inescapable" to the therapist, the therapist is exercising
choice and discretion about the timing and content of specific
disclosures made. More about that later. On the other hand,
"inadvertent self-disclosure" feels to the analyst and patient as
if it pops out of the therapist's psyche spontaneously, even
suddenly, in the midst of evocative interactive process. Such
inadvertent self-disclosure—which may be a quip, slip, a
flash of fear or temper, a retort, or an exclamation—often
feels as if the therapist has just stumbled upon the tip of an
iceberg, and latent transference—countertransference positions, or some relational dilemma slow-cooking over time is
now flushed out into the room of potential reflection. We find
a perfect example of this in Strean, when Bella, the wrestler,
threatens "to beat the shit" out of him and asks him if he is
scared. "Quivering, I said spontaneously, 'I'm scared shitless.
You can beat me up and I think you will.'" At this, the tip of
the iceberg melted. "[S]he put down the chair and said 'I'm
proud of you, Herby!' and shook my hand." Now the work
would begin. But what defines the work? Bella's character?
The impasse? Or her therapist's inadvertent disclosure? Inadvertent self-disclosure is an inevitable outcome of the analyst's
engagement with a patient. It cuts across diagnosis. I would

add that with patients who want a minimum of responsiveness because they need a maximum of space, the analyst must
pay particular attention to inadvertent disclosures in nonverbal form, lapses of attention, empathic failures, or slips. Such
self-disclosures may or may not contain within them elements
from the analyst's life experience. The responsible clinician,
with appropriate caution and respect for the power inherent
in any self-disclosure on her part, must be prepared for this
inevitable eventuality. Inadvertent self-disclosure requires,
above all else, the therapist's skill in utilizing the potential of
the shared contents of her experience in the service of the
therapeutic process.

The dimension of self-disclosure that I call "deliberate" is
the therapist's sharing of some personal material or personal
process, whether it be an association, a way of thinking about
the patient that *names* countertransference rather than inter-
preting the transference, an anecdote, or a personal perspective on the challenges of living. Consider, for example, Strean's
revealing to his abused patient, Amy, that *he* felt helpless, and
later in the treatment his paradoxical statement that he would
have loved to have a daughter like her. In the clinical process
there are times when the patient is ready to take in some
elements from the therapist's subjectivity. When the patient
appears to be feeling empty or "drawing a blank," she is
sometimes, in effect, asking the therapist to provide something that is "other than me" (see Winnicott 1969) to open up
an area that the therapist's silence may not supply (Pizer
1997).

A final statement of the obvious about all three dimensions of disclosure. It is inappropriate to suggest a specific
recipe for the when and how of disclosure in the consulting
room. As clinicians, how and when we advertently choose to
communicate to our patients is inextricably linked to who we
are, our technical framework, our personal boundaries, beliefs, and sense of comfort. This is particularly important
since, whatever we say to our patients, we remain responsible

for our revelations as we consider every subsequent interaction in the life of that particular treatment. What I mean by responsibility (and here I include inadvertent disclosure as well) is the effort to remain alert to the repercussions of shared personal material in the same spirit that we attempt to follow the development of our patients' material. Furthermore, as in the case of inescapable and deliberate disclosure, it is critical to consider our current affective state before we attempt to communicate to a patient our awareness of an uninvited elephant. As I said in my article, "Not every therapist with breast cancer would make the personal choice to disclose her condition to her patients. *Nor should she.* Among the many personal issues one may or may not choose to share with a patient, cancer is an intensely personal matter. . . . Thus, each analyst must remain attentive and connected to her own sense of how stable she can remain in the face of uncertainties, how grounded and prepared she is to deal with whatever surprises of affect or inquiry may arise" (Pizer 1997, pp. 454–455).

The late David Feinsilver wrote a paper (1998) about the therapeutic action entailed in telling all of his patients that he was dying of metastatic colon cancer. He wanted them to be among the first to know. In that paper he presented three clinical vignettes of his disclosure to patients from across the diagnostic spectrum, attempting to demonstrate the therapeutic importance of disclosure. Answering his own question as to whether or not his disclosure to patients had a mobilizing effect, he noted that aspects of his illness were both perceived and misperceived, regardless of what he chose to say to them. He wrote:

> This would correspond with what Pizer (1997) calls an "inescapable disclosure" as opposed to a "deliberate disclosure." The therapeutic importance of a disclosure is not just that it reveals something previously unknown or hidden, but whether or not it

begins deliberately to bring ego resources to an issue that is potentially threatening because of its being present either inadvertently, or inescapably, as "an elephant in the room." Threatening inescapable or inadvertent disclosures thus become transformed into useful deliberate disclosures. This promotes the alliance. [p. 1143]

But what about the transference? How many times have the therapy police warned us that by drawing attention to ourselves we become guilty of disturbing the transference! Here we need to pause a moment to consider what Feinsilver has suggested. He cuts across diagnostic categories and illustrates how our overlapping inventory of disclosures moves and merges toward deliberate disclosure, which, he believes, promotes the therapeutic alliance. The implication here indeed might be that, for the most part, not to disclose would constitute some kind of break. But let us continue with the development of his thesis. Feinsilver writes "[A] disclosure can either be threatening or reassuring depending on whether or not it is done in a way that maximizes ego-mastery and limits fantasy. What is important about disclosure is not simply that it divulge something but that it helps to re-establish *the dialectical balance* between being analytic and being supportive" (p. 1143, author's emphasis).

And so, with this conclusion, I hope I have adequately responded to Herbert Strean's request for further research as well as a response to his paper. I'm willing to bet that we have, in fact, met in the middle, but still not, to my chagrin, in person.

REFERENCES

Feinsilver, D. B. (1998). The therapist as a person facing death: the hardest of external realities and therapeutic action. *International Journal of Psycho-Analysis* 79:1131–1150.

Pizer, B. (1997). When the analyst is ill: dimensions of self-disclosure. *Psychoanalytic Quarterly* 66:450–469.

Winnicott, D. W. (1969). The use of an object and relating through identifications. In *Playing and Reality*, pp. 86–94. New York: Basic Books, 1971.

Discussion:
Engaging Patients
Authentically

Martha Stark

Herbert Strean has written a compelling paper in which he persuasively speaks to the effectiveness of countertransference disclosure in resolving certain therapeutic impasses. It is unusual to find someone so open to sharing the intimate details of what goes on in his consulting room. The clinical vignettes Strean offers demonstrate convincingly how the therapist's selective disclosure of his countertransference, by introducing aspects of his authentic self, enables patient and therapist to find each other in a more deeply personal way and thereby facilitates resolution of the therapeutic impasse.

I could not agree more heartily with Strean's basic premise that resolving a stuck place may require of the therapist that he participate as not simply an observer but as a participant-observer. Indeed, working with such a two-person model of therapeutic action may be exactly what is needed for patient and therapist to be able to break out of what has become an otherwise intractably deadlocked situation.

As I was reading and rereading Strean's case examples, however, I found myself thinking about how the deadlocked situations he describes had developed in the first place. The therapeutic impasses may arise because Strean, despite his belief in a two-person model, for the most part, seems to me to embrace a one-person model of therapeutic action in which he posits insight and enhancement of the patient's knowledge as the primary therapeutic goals. In every one of his five examples, Strean's aim appears to be to help the patient gain a deeper understanding of his unconscious process and therefore more insight into the internal workings of his mind. To that end, I suggest that Strean offers the patient experience-distant interpretations intended to render conscious the patient's unconscious.

With Amy, for example, Strean tells us that his interventions were "designed to weaken her punitive superego and give her permission to own her own rage." He interpreted to Amy that he thought she was "having difficulty feeling her hurt and anger toward her grandfather and mother." Instead of responding by acknowledging just how angry she was at them, she responded by directing her anger toward herself, protesting that had she been a more "decent person," not as "disgusting," she would not have been beaten in the first place and would now have a good job and a decent man in her life. Then when Strean attempted to "help her see that she was punishing herself for her strong hostile and erotic fantasies," Amy ignored that intervention entirely and "avoided" him. It was only when Strean shared with Amy his countertransference reaction of outrage (about her grandfather's raping her and her mother's complicity in it) that Amy was able to experience him as actually caring. But, after another two months, Amy was once again experiencing Strean as not caring very much about her. Although he notes (to the reader) that he thought Amy had become "very paranoid," I was wondering if, indeed, he had once again stepped back and positioned himself outside the therapeutic field, the better to observe Amy and formulate hypotheses about her internal process, but a stance that was making Amy experience him as more distant, less a participant, more an observer. In other words, perhaps Amy's "paranoid" reaction to Strean was at least in part the result of his shifting from a more involved two-person to a more detached one-person therapeutic posture—perhaps all the more confusing for Amy in light of Strean's earlier heartfelt disclosure of his countertransference reaction of outrage on her behalf.

A two-person conceptualization of the therapeutic process would have it that both the therapist's countertransference (about which I will be saying more a little later) and the patient's transference are co-created, co-constructed, co-determined—that is, a story about both participants in the therapeutic dyad. In other words, Amy's transference experience of Strean as no longer caring about her might not be just a "paranoid" distortion (and a story about her abusive early object relationships) but also a legitimate response to Strean's once again less disclosing, more interpretive, more distant stance. A two-person perspective would have it that therapists should be ever open to recognizing what Greenberg (1991) has referred to as the "realistic" aspects of the patient's negative transference. If, indeed, Amy's experience of Strean is at least in part her reaction to his retreat from a two-person, participant-observer stance to a more one-person, observer stance, then it is not entirely fair for Strean to be thinking that the "problem" is entirely Amy's (in the form of her being "very paranoid"). Rather, it behooves him to take seriously her commentary and to hold himself more accountable for the part he might have played in her experience of him as not caring.

When, at this point, Strean offers Amy an experience-distant interpretation that aims to help her understand more about her contribution to the negative transference ("I tried to show her that she was afraid to trust me or feel intimate toward me"), Amy, I believe somewhat understandably, is not all that interested and responds by insisting that he is a "phony." But when Strean shares with Amy his countertransference reaction of helplessness and upset about her "constantly labeling me a phony," Amy welcomes his "authenticity" and even begins to develop sexual feelings about him.

Although I know Herb to be a wonderfully warm, emotionally present, refreshingly unaffected, unusually humble man with a delightful sense of humor, it would seem that in his work with Amy (as with the others), the position he assumes is much more that of an authority than that of a collaborator. In other words, his stance is that of a classically trained psychoanalytic clinician whose primary goal, it would seem, is to pass along to Amy his formulations about the internal workings of her mind, so that she can come to know as much about her unconscious process as he does. This posture reminds me of something Lacan (1977) once wrote— namely, that in a classical psychoanalysis, the patient gets better once the patient has come to know all that the analyst knows which is what the patient had unconsciously known all along!

That Amy was initially "shocked" when Strean disclosed some of his positive countertransference reactions (saying that he would "love to have a daughter like her") suggests to me that he may well have felt all kinds of warm and loving feelings toward her but did not reveal them to her as much as he could and, perhaps, should have. I am anticipating that Strean might respond by saying that Amy's shock was truly much more a story about her difficulty tolerating intimacy than about his not having revealed to her his positive feelings about her. But it would at least have been worth considering what his contribution might have been to Amy's negative experience of him as not caring. Interestingly, and not unexpectedly, once Amy developed a strong therapeutic alliance with Strean, she found herself wanting "stories that demonstrated how much I loved her."

Apparently, once the therapeutic impasses between them were worked through, Amy and Strean went on to do some very fine work over the course of the next three and a half years. Although it is hard to imagine that Amy could have advanced from being a "lowly secretary" (at the beginning of their time together) to being a "very successful instructor in a leading university" (four years later), it would seem that by virtue of Strean's ability to make judicious use of both his negative and his positive countertransference responses to her, was indeed able to make some very impressive gains in her life and in the treatment. It is also of note that Amy, after four years, is doing a "great deal of constructive self-examination and analyzing her transference reactions with much creativity and enthusiasm." I would simply add, at this point, that were Strean to embrace, more generally, a two-person model of therapeutic action in which he recognized his ongoing participation as a participant observer with his own subjectivity (and not just an objectively detached observer), then he as well would be engaged in constructive and creative self-examination and would be willing to look at his own contribution to Amy's negative perceptions of him (as well as his own contribution to the negative countertransference that he develops toward Amy).

It is fortunate that Strean not only was able to recognize the importance of letting himself be found by way of selectively disclosing his countertransference reactions but was also courageous enough to deliver himself in this way into the relationship. Indeed, each time he dared to share some of what he was feeling toward Amy (whether positive or negative), she responded by opening up more.

Generally, I believe that a two-person, relational approach, from beginning to end, and not just at those times when a therapeutic impasse has arisen, can foster development of a strong positive alliance, thereby creating a space within which the patient, of her own accord and at her own pace, can arrive at a more intimate understanding of her internal process, but only when she has signaled that she is ready. When, however, the focus is more interpretive from the start, the potential is there for the development of a therapeutic impasse, in which the patient experiences both that she has not been found and that she has not been able to find the therapist. A therapist who offers experience-distant interpretations to a patient who is not sure she yet dares to bring her authentic self into the relationship may actually be contributing to the development of a negative transference or even a therapeutic impasse.

I am suggesting, then, that were Strean to have delivered more of his real self into the relationship from the start, Amy might not have experienced him as uncaring, unauthentic. It is important, however, not to lose sight of the fact that had Strean not failed her in the ways that he did, then inevitably (and necessarily) he would have failed her in other ways, because a truly relational perspective has it that the patient who suffered childhood trauma (1) has a need to be now failed by her present objects as she was once failed by her past objects and, therefore, (2) exerts interpersonal pressure on them to so fail her.

As with all repetition compulsions, part of a patient's need to be failed has an unhealthy component (it is, after all, more comfortable, less anxiety-provoking, to experience something so familiar, no matter how pathological, because this is the only way the patient knows to engage her objects) and a healthy component (there is the desire to achieve belated mastery). Consequently, it is not only inevitable but necessary and even desirable that the patient eventually succeed in getting her therapist to fail her in ways specifically determined by her developmental history, so that she can at last work through and master her internal demons, thereby securing a better outcome this time. Greenberg (1986) has suggested that if the therapist does not participate as a new object, the therapy never gets under way; if he does not participate as the old one, the therapy never ends—which captures exquisitely the delicate balance between the therapist's participation as a new good object (so that there can be a starting over or a new beginning) and the therapist's participation as the old bad object (so that there can be a reworking of internalized traumas).

In the case of Bella, here too Strean appears to understand her internal dynamics and attempts to communicate this understanding to her by way of interpretations designed to enhance her self-knowledge. As an example, he says that it was clear to him the day he met Bella that, "as a product of a broken family, she used her strong, aggressive demeanor as a defense to ward off feelings of closeness and vulnerability."

In marked contrast to this is the contemporary, two-person conception of the truth as always relative, subjective, and unknowable. Because there is no absolute truth that is objectively real, the therapist must be able to tolerate the anxiety of not knowing for sure and the necessary uncertainty that is at the heart of the therapeutic process.

Strean, however, tells us that he offered Bella "interpretations suggesting that she wanted to defeat me, scare me." He acknowledges that these (experience-distant) formulations "got nowhere." I have the sense, however, that he attributed the failure of his intervention more to her (and her inability/unwillingness to recognize the "truth" in what he was saying) than to him (perhaps inaccurate content, perhaps poor timing, perhaps provocative delivery). Here, as with Amy, interpretations were offered by someone positioned outside the therapeutic field, formulating hypotheses about what he thought were underlying motivations.

Bella, understandably, was not particularly open to his efforts to heighten the level of her awareness about her desire to frighten him. When Strean later tells Bella that he thought she wanted to "get me very angry at her and put me in a fighting mood," he was once again embracing a one-person psychology, presuming that he was in the know and wanting to convey that knowledge to Bella. Bella responded with mockery, contempt, and outrage, even threatening to "beat the shit out of [him]" with a chair she had just grabbed.

A relational model would understand Bella's experience

of Strean as "a weak fairy" who "could not help a soul" as co-created, that is, as a story about both patient (and her need to experience her therapist as helpless, scared, and weak) and therapist (and his actual participation as a helpless, scared, and weak man). In other words, if the patient develops a negative transference, a relational perspective would have it that the patient's negative feelings about the therapist are not just attributable to her "distorted" perceptions of him; rather, there may well also be a component of her negative feelings about him that speaks to his contribution to that experience (earlier referred to as the realistic aspects of the transference). Although Strean courageously acknowledges his fear when Bella threatens to hit him with the chair, prior to that, he does not appear to recognize any "truth" in Bella's description of him as helpless and weak.

Bella tells Strean, "If you had told me earlier in the game that you were furious with me, we could have had a better dialogue." In essence, Bella is suggesting that had Strean been more comfortable with a two-person, interactive model from the beginning, then perhaps they could have had a more meaningful, more mutual exchange from that point forward.

Strean makes an important observation in his discussion of his work with Bella. At one point in the treatment, Bella notes, "I got you to express all of the terror that I was unwilling to express. Now I seem freer to be myself with you." She was indeed then able to give voice to her own fear, once Strean had been able to give voice to his. Casement (1985) writes about the patient's use of "communication by impact" to convey the unspeakable to his therapist. According to Casement, there is interactional pressure, the unconscious intent of which is to make the therapist have feelings the patient must disavow. It is the therapist's ability to tolerate the intolerable that makes the patient's previously unmanageable feelings more manageable for him.

My own experience has been that there are some patients who cannot tolerate having feelings like shame, hatred, envy, or love in the presence of another until they have managed to elicit in the other those very feelings. For example, one of my patients could deliver her shame into our relationship only after she had managed to provoke my own shame; she could bring her tears into the room only after she had finally brought me to tears. Her grief became less terrifying by virtue of the fact that I was able to carry that grief on her behalf. For my patient to be alone with her feelings was intolerable, but once she knew that I had become as vulnerable as she was, she could dare to be more affectively present—she could dare to feel.

At this point, I would like to speak to another issue raised by Strean's paper—namely, the role of intentionality on the patient's part. I conceptualize interpersonally provocative behavior on the patient's part as an enactment, the intent of which, even if unconscious, is to elicit a particular response from the therapist—perhaps a response that is familiar, even if pathological, because that may be the only way the patient knows how to engage the other. In fact, I believe that the concept of enactment is an extremely useful construct in a relational model because it conceives of the patient as intentioned in his actions, that is, as intent upon either eliciting a particular response from the therapist or conveying to the therapist something deeply important about his internal world.

In Strean's five vignettes, he speaks to the impact his patients' behaviors have on him, but, for the most part, he does not appear to consider that his patients might have needed to provoke a particular response from him. With Bella, he does speak to her desire to "get me very angry at her" and to "put me in a fighting mood," although he does not speak to the issue of why she might have had such a desire. And with Charlie, he does suggest that "the only thing you want is to fight with me," although here too he does not speak to the issue of why he might have been trying to provoke a fight.

My own belief, as I noted earlier, is that the patient who was traumatized as a child will, under the sway of the repetition compulsion, be intent upon re-creating the early-on traumatic failure situation in the here-and-now engagement with his therapist, and the patient's provocative enactments are intended (even if unconsciously) to do just this, so that he can master the trauma.

Because a relational perspective is an intersubjective one involving two authentic subjects in relationship, not only the patient's subjectivity but also the therapist's subjectivity (and its impact on the patient) must be taken into consideration when considering the experience of each participant in the dyad.

Interestingly, whereas Bella told Strean she thought he was a "weak fairy" who "could not help a soul," so too Charlie came to experience Strean as a "weak sister who can't take it." If only one patient experiences the therapist in a certain way, then it may well be primarily a story about the patient. But if two or more patients experience the therapist in the same way, then it behooves the therapist to think about whether there is something in what he is doing that would lead his patients to experience him in that way. With respect to Strean, it would be important for him to consider why some of his patients experience him as weak and ineffectual and as someone who can be mocked and treated contemptuously.

I believe that a therapist who embraces a primarily interpretive, more classical model of therapeutic action will indeed run the risk of being experienced by the patient as weak and ineffectual, as not authentic and not caring. In other words, this may be the price a therapist pays for being somewhat authoritarian in the delivery of his experience-distant interpretations and for being more revealing, vulnerable, and genuine only in the aftermath of a therapeutic impasse.

Paralleling Winnicott's (1965) distinction between the subjective countertransference (a story about the therapist) and the objective countertransference (a story about the patient and the patient's impact on the therapist), elsewhere I have made the distinction (Stark 1999) between the subjective transference (a story about the patient) and the objective transference (a story about the therapist and the therapist's impact on the patient). In other words, just as the objective countertransference is what any therapist, were he to be honest with himself, would experience in relation to the patient, so, too, the objective transference is what any patient, were he to be honest with himself, would feel in response to the therapist.

I believe that it behooves all of us to think about the ways our patients tend to experience us, particularly when they are angry with us. In other words, what kind of impact do we tend to have on our patients? The response we tend to elicit may be either because of the approach we take or, more generally, who we are (our subjectivity).

Every therapist has some kind of impact. He could be experienced as warm, loving, empathic, responsive, protective, concerned or more removed, detached, not available, intellectual, critical. Some therapists are experienced as fragile, narcissistically vulnerable, insecure; some therapists appear to be made anxious by the patient's anger; some therapists are felt to be demanding, insistent, pressuring, expectant, opinionated. I have a colleague who is fairly consistently seen by her patients as being in the enviable position of "having it all"; another friend of mine is experienced by many of their as having difficulty with his patients' terminations. Rather than positively and negatively valenced attributes, each therapist brings his likes, dislikes, preferences, fears, needs, strengths, idiosyncrasies. We must always remember that our patients are every bit as busy sizing us up as we are sizing them up—and some of their perceptions may indeed be uncannily on target.

This is all by way of saying that I believe the responses we tend to elicit from our patients (in essence, the objective transference) are usually as much a story about us as they are about the patient and that we must take seriously our patients' protests, objections, and negative commentaries. In other words, since we are the common denominator, the patient's response may well be more a story about us than a story about him.

Elsewhere (Stark 1994a,b) I suggest that the therapist, moment by moment, must decide whether he wants to be with the patient where the patient is or he wants to direct the patient's attention elsewhere. In the first instance, he will be helping the patient to gain understanding; in the second instance, he will be helping the patient to feel understood. Experience-distant interventions are designed to enhance the patient's knowledge; experience-near interventions are designed to validate the patient's experience. There are benefits and risks to each stance. My point here is that it is important for each of us to be aware of how our choice in this regard will have a major impact on how our patients will tend to experience us.

One of the inherent problems with an approach that places a premium on the therapist's enhancement of the patient's knowledge by way of thoughtfully formulated interpretations is that when the patient challenges the authority of the therapist or the correctness of his interventions, the therapist may well experience it as a narcissistic injury, reacting with upset, hurt, anger. In fact, it would seem that many of Strean's countertransference disclosures involve his sharing of angry, injured, frustrated, hurt feelings with patients who seem to have provoked such feelings by being relatively non-responsive to, or even dismissive of, Strean's efforts to advance their understanding of themselves. More generally, when a therapist is very invested in helping his patients get better, he will be more at risk for developing negative countertransference. In Strean's own words, "Because I genuinely wanted to help these patients but found that my efforts to do so were strongly opposed, I reacted with

feelings of hurt, frustration, irritation, alienation, helplessness, boredom, revenge, or with a combination of these
feelings." I believe that all of us therapists are prone to these
feelings in response to narcissistic blows we receive from our
patients; it behooves us to beware of being too invested in
helping our patients to get better (whatever "getting better"
might mean!) because such pressure may not be helpful and
may, instead, create the potential for a power struggle or a
therapeutic impasse.

Whenever the therapist finds himself feeling frustrated,
hurt, impatient, annoyed, injured, it is crucial that he be
willing to look at that part of his countertransference response that may be subjective, that is, what he brings from his
own history to the interaction. In other words, although a
provocative patient will probably provoke any therapist, the
particular form that the therapist's countertransference reaction takes may be as much about the therapist and his own
vulnerabilities as it is about the patient's provocative enactment. It would be important for Strean and for all who dare
to write about their countertransference responses to be
willing to examine the contribution of their own subjectivity
to their reactivity to the patient.

Strean concludes his discussion with the following: "I
believe that disclosing of the countertransference when there
is a therapeutic impasse helps keep the patient in treatment
and helps the therapist want to continue working with the
patient." I would like to conclude my discussion of Strean's
courageous, thought-provoking paper with the thought that
making use of the therapist's countertransference, more generally, helps keep the patient in treatment and helps the
therapist want to continue working with the patient.

I believe that if the therapist does not bring his authentic
self into the room, then the patient may end up analyzed, but
never reached. If the therapist does not allow himself to
become a participant in what unfolds between them, then the
patient may end up a lot wiser than when he started, but still

not found. By using his countertransference, the therapist is able to find, and to be found by, the patient.

I believe that although Strean is, everything considered, more naturally a one-person than a two-person therapist, he was nonetheless able to go where he needed to go and to do what he needed to do when the occasion called for it. His paper is an important contribution to the literature on countertransference disclosure. It is not the final word (nor is it intended to be), but it definitely advances our understanding of the role played by the therapist's use of his countertransference to engage his patients authentically in the therapy relationship.

REFERENCES

Casement, P. (1985). Forms of interactive communication. In *On Learning from the Patient*, pp. 72–101. London and New York: Tavistock.

Greenberg, J. (1986). Theoretical models and the analyst's neutrality. *Contemporary Psychoanalysis* 22:87–106.

——— (1991). Countertransference and reality. *Psychoanalytic Dialogues* 1(1):52–73.

Lacan, J. (1977). *Ecrits: A Selection*. New York: Norton.

Stark, M. (1994a). *Working with Resistance*. Northvale, NJ: Jason Aronson.

——— (1994b). *A Primer on Working with Resistance*. Northvale, NJ: Jason Aronson.

——— (1999). *Modes of Therapeutic Action: Enhancement of Knowledge, Provision of Experience, and Engagement in Relationship*. Northvale, NJ: Jason Aronson.

Winnicott, D. W. (1965). *The Maturational Processes and the Facilitating Environment*. New York: International Universities Press.

5

Resolving Therapeutic Impasses by Using the Supervisor's Countertransference

A little over four decades ago when I was a supervisor at a treatment institution for emotionally disturbed youngsters, I was summoned one day to the director's office. Without warning, I was told that as part of the process of being groomed to be his assistant director, I would be required to fire one of my supervisees. Very anxious, extremely self-conscious, and most uncertain about how I would conduct myself, after much hesitation I arranged an appointment with my supervisee. With enormous trepidation, I initiated the discussion by asking, "How is it going, Melvin?" To my deep consternation, Melvin confidently and enthusiastically responded, "I think you're doing a good job!"

Although Melvin's reply to my query might be considered somewhat unconventional even in the year 2001, it was out of this world in 1959. Forty years ago a supervisee was almost always deferential to his supervisor and hardly ever made evaluative remarks about her. He did what he was told without ever questioning the directive, as I behaved when my supervisor told me to fire Melvin.

From the inception of social work practice and through the early 1960s, supervision was essentially an administrative function (Richmond 1917, Williamson 1965). In essence, the practitioner was directed to fulfill the mission of the agency by practicing what the supervisor preached. The agency prescribed how the social worker should function on the job, and the supervisor tried her best to ensure that the agency's mandates would be executed faithfully by the supervisee. Although the administrative role of the supervisor has not disappeared and is particularly present in today's mental health centers and other social agencies, many increments have been made to the role set of the clinical supervisor during the last four decades. By the 1960s the supervisor had a teaching function (Feldman 1950). In addition to ensuring that the supervisee was adapting to the agency's policies, she helped the practitioner learn to make more sophisticated diagnostic assessments, devise more creative treatment plans, and integrate salient practice principles (Bibring 1950). As notions like transference, countertransference, resistance, and psychogenesis became very much in vogue in mental health parlance, not only was the clinician helped to study the unconscious meaning of his interactions with clients, but his transference reactions and resistances to his mentor were also subjects for study within the supervisory process (Fleming and Benedek 1966).

Searles (1955, 1962) was one of the first to discuss how supervisory interaction was influenced by transference and countertransference interaction in the treatment relationship. He suggested that clarifying the problems the practitioner experienced in the supervision would not only diminish the resistances to learning but would also foster change in the therapy. Ekstein and Wallerstein (1972) also discussed this parallel process and delineated ways in which it could be used to understand the therapeutic atmosphere. They focused on the supervisee's inevitable problems about learning (interpersonal problems between supervisor and supervisee and the supervisee's resistance to supervision) in order to clarify the transference–countertransference problems between therapist and patient.

In 1966 Fleming and Benedek contributed the concept of the *learning alliance* in supervision. This notion parallels that of the *therapeutic alliance* (Greenson 1967) and was viewed as the basis of trust, shared learning goals, and mutual involvement on which supervision should be grounded. Doehrman (1976) substantiated empirically the Ekstein and Wallerstein (1972) concept of *parallel process of supervision*. She demonstrated that difficulties in the therapeutic relationship were unconsciously communicated to the supervisor by the way the practitioner interacted with his mentor. Unexpectedly, she found that the influence of the supervisor's emotional reactions to the supervisee and to the patient were an outstanding feature of the processes observed.

THE SUPERVISOR'S ANONYMITY

Until quite recently, descriptions of supervision that recognize that both supervisor and supervisee mutually influence one another in the supervisory process have only rarely been found in the mental health literature (Lane 1990, Rock 1997). As Rock (1997) has stated: "Reports from supervisees about their personal experience in supervision are few and far between, while reports from supervisors about their private experience of the work as opposed to their prescriptions and proscriptions, observations and formulations are even harder to find. Searles's early papers on supervision (1955, 1962) are remarkable exceptions to this observation in that they demonstrate the great value to the student of supervision of disclosure of the inner experience of the supervisor" (p. 4).

For many decades, both within social work and among

its allied professions, when conflict developed within the supervisory relationship it was generally believed that it was emanating from the supervisee (Teitelbaum 1990). The underlying assumption was that the more experienced, better trained (and usually better analyzed) supervisor was less responsible for supervisory problems than was her less experienced and less aware supervisee.

A good example of how supervision was traditionally conducted in the mental health professions was presented by Greenson (1967). He described how a supervisee of his in order to appear neutral, abstinent, and anonymous, maintained his silence after his patient expressed extreme distress over the sudden and serious illness of her infant son. In response to the supervisee's remarks that the patient's tears and subsequent silence "represented a resistance," Greenson noted, "I shook my head in disbelief and I ended the session by telling him that his emotional unresponsiveness would prevent the formation of a working alliance. . . . I then suggested that he might benefit from some further analysis" (p. 220). Greenson concluded his vignette with an admonition: "These clinical data demonstrate the fact that an objectionable trait in the analyst can produce realistic reactions in the patient which preclude successful psychoanalytic treatment" (p. 221). What Greenson omitted from his account were his own countertransference reactions to the patient and his supervisee. It may be hypothesized that Greenson was very identified with the patient's pain and sense of vulnerability and concomitantly felt punitive toward the supervisee, who did not overtly empathize with the patient. Unaware of his countertransference reactions, Greenson helped create a parallel process in the supervision whereby the supervisee's failure to empathize with his patient was recaptitulated by the supervisor's failure to empathize with the supervisee.

That the impact of the supervisor's contertransference reactions to her supervisee and his patient was seldom addressed in the mental health literature is not too surprising. It is similar to the history of what has been emphasized and deemphasized in studying the psychotherapeutic relationship. In contrast to his comprehensive and meticulous discussions of transference (1912, 1914, 1915, 1926), the founder of modern psychotherapy, Sigmund Freud, wrote very little on the subject of countertransference. As Abend (1980) has pointed out, "Freud's original idea that countertransference means unconscious interference with [a therapist's] ability to understand patients has been broadened during the past forty years: current usage often includes all of the emotional reactions at work" (p. 374).

Just as the earlier clinicians had little to say about countertransference and did not view the therapist's subjectivity as a central component of the treatment, likewise in supervision, until recently, only limited consideration has been given to the effects of the supervisor's unresolved conflicts, blind spots, inappropriate expectations, or what Teitelbaum (1990) refers to as the *supertransference*.

Similar to the literature on failures in psychotherapy that has focused almost exclusively on the patient's responsibility with limited attention given to the therapist's contributions (Chessick 1971, Strean 1986, Wolman 1972), misalliances in the supervisory relationship have largely been attributed to the supervisee. As a result, the authoritarian atmosphere noted earlier in the Greenson example was for many decades par for the course of supervision. In the available literature on supervision it would appear the rule rather than the exception that the supervisor would take over the case, point out how she would deal with the material, and try to get the supervisee to imitate her (Fleming and Benedek 1966).

The type of supervision practiced for many decades in social work and elsewhere has been aptly termed *superego training* (Balint 1948, Fine 1990). It consisted of what Glover (1952) called "authoritarian spoon feeding, a mid-Victorian pedagogy." This form of supervision fostered excessive dependency on the supervisor (Arlow 1963), squelched the supervisee's autonomy, and made it difficult for him to become a creative practitioner.

THE SUPERVISOR COMES OUT OF THE CLOSET

Although as early as 1954 Benedek called attention to the importance of unresolved problems in the supervisor as a factor contributing toward negative therapeutic outcomes, twenty-five years later Langs (1979) concluded, "There has been a rather striking neglect in the literature of the supervisor's countertransference and . . . it deserves systematic consideration" (p. 333). Later, Schlesinger (1981) echoed the sentiment and suggested that the supervisor may unwittingly contribute to the supervisee's learning problems and the patient's eventual lack of progress in treatment. In 1984 Issacharoff dealt somewhat more directly with the supervisor's countertransference issues, pointing out how the latter may enact a role of overprotective parent, overly critical parent, or both. The supervisee, treated like a weak and/or disappointing son or daughter, may then act out with his or her patient in the therapy the anger and discomfort stimulated in supervision.

Just as most therapy patients and their practitioners have the potential to collude with each other to gratify certain illusions of the patient, such as the latter's yearning to be the therapist's favorite child, or to symbiose with the therapist and become omnipotent like the therapist appears to be, similar illusions can be present in the teaching–learning situation in which supervisor and supervisee can also collude. Supervisee and supervisor can share the illusion that the supervisor is omniscient whereas the supervisee and patient know next to nothing. They can suffer together from the illusion that the supervisor is exempt from pathology, ignorance, and blind spots, whereas the supervisee and the patient are both struggling to maintain their sanity. The learner and his mentor can delude themselves into believing that the supervisor's sexual and aggressive fantasies are in superb control whereas the patient and the supervisee are either too inhibited by their punitive superegos or too expressive because of their superego lacunae (Teitelbaum 1990).

As Lesser (1984) noted, certain illusions may exist in supervision such as "the supervisor is always objective" or "the supervisor always knows best." She further pointed out that the supervisor's anxieties are "generally unrecognized, perhaps because anxieties are less acceptable to the supervisor than to the supervisee. Yet, awareness of the supervisor's anxieties is essential for fulfilling the supervisory task" (p. 147).

As the aforementioned citations suggest, just as psychotherapeutic interventions by the practitioner are always an expression of his countertransference even when the technical procedure is considered to be valid and acceptable (Jacobs 1986) so, too, can the supervisor's responses be colored by supertransference (Teitelbaum 1990). As more practitioners are shifting their conceptualization of countertransference from the traditional classical model of a one-person psychology nearer to a two-person psychology, it is now a virtual axiom that the therapist's countertransference and the patient's transference always influence both parties and, therefore, always affect the therapeutic outcome. Now, the same notion can and is being made about supervision—both parties affect each other and both contribute to the supervisory outcome (Lane 1990, Rock 1997, Strean 1991, 1999, Teitelbaum 1990).

In a previous paper (Strean 1999) I attempted to demonstrate how certain therapeutic impasses can be resolved when the therapist shares some of his countertransference reactions with the patient. I suggested that the disclosure of the therapist's countertransference frequently tends to clarify the patient's transference. In addition, by the therapist's appearing less authoritarian, more egalitarian and authentic when sharing his inner processes, it was demonstrated that clients were then more enabled to share their feelings, fantasies, and memories in the treatment. Inasmuch as therapeutic impasses frequently involve a lot of unexpressed hostility, the therapist's disclosing his countertransference responses tended to help the patient discharge her hostility and feel safer and less antagonistic in the therapy. As I witnessed the resolution of many treatment impasses both in my own practice as well as in those of my colleagues and supervisees, I decided to take the use of self-disclosure of the countertransference one step further. In those cases where my supervisee and I were not witnessing much therapeutic movement, I shared certain selected countertransference reactions with the supervisee that I was experiencing toward his patients, toward him, and toward their interaction.

In the remaining part of this chapter, I will discuss several therapeutic impasses that moved toward resolution when I shared some of my countertransference responses with my supervisees. I will also attempt to explain why disclosure of the supervisor's countertransference can, at crucial times, resolve treatment impasses that other supervisory interventions do not achieve. However, before doing so I would like to offer a few comments on the modern supervisor's complex role set.

THE COMPLEX ROLE SET OF THE
CLINICAL SUPERVISOR

The evolution of the role set of the supervisor has paralleled the professional development of the clinician. Just as the contemporary therapist has moved from his conceptualization of the treatment situation from a one-person to a two-person interaction, the supervisor has reformulated her notion of supervision in a similar manner. And, just as the modern therapist no longer sees himself as a blank screen but is subject to the patient's transference reactions and his own countertransferences and counterresistances, the supervisor has moved from the exclusive position of teacher, administrator, and overseer to being what Marshall (1997) has formulated: "[The modern supervisor] is now an integral part of a system wherein [she] is influenced not only by the therapist, patient and [her] own promptings, but is a prime source of feedback to the patient through the supervisee" (p. 77). The contemporary supervisor still retains her teaching function but as she helps her supervisee enhance his diagnostic thinking and refine his therapeutic interventions, she constantly considers how she is being experienced by the supervisee and how his transference reactions toward her stimulate or inhibit his learning. Today, the supervisor makes an educational diagnosis of her supervisee, determines with him what he needs to learn and what his learning capacities and limitations are (Rock 1997). Just as the therapist has to decide with the client when and how to support her, when and what to clarify or interpret, the supervisor has to determine with the supervisee what will be most beneficial to the supervisee at a particular time with a particular patient (Strean 1991, Teitelbaum 1990).

Not only does the supervisor have to deal with her countertransference reactions to the supervisee but she also has to cope with her countertransference toward the supervisee's client. In some ways the supervisee's client becomes the supervisor's client! Therefore, the supervisor must consistently be aware of the fantasies, memories, and anxieties that the supervisee's client activates in her. Of enormous importance, the supervisor also has to understand her countertransference responses to the interaction between the supervisee and his client. Does she feel like a competitive lover? An overprotective parent? A jealous child? Perhaps all of the above?

Until now, virtually all of the literature on the supervisor's countertransference reactions has implied that the supervisor understands her responses but keeps them to herself. I intend to demonstrate how the supervisor's sharing of certain countertransference responses with the supervisee can resolve therapeutic impasses and strengthen the therapeutic alliance between the supervisee and his client. Just as I believe that the therapist's disclosures of countertransference reactions to the patient can at crucial times strengthen the therapeutic alliance, I also contend that the supervisor's disclosures of her countertransference responses can strengthen the supervisory alliance. In my judgment, when the supervisory alliance is strengthened, the therapeutic alliance between the patient and the therapist is strengthened, thereby moving the treatment relationship toward a resolution of the therapeutic impasse.

The following section presents several short vignettes that involve therapeutic impasses that supervisees of mine were experiencing with specific clients, and that were not being resolved through supervision. I will describe the nature of the impasse, review what transpired in supervision but did not help resolve the impasse, state the specific content of my countertransference disclosure, and describe the supervisee's response to my disclosure. Finally, I will discuss the client's response after the supervisee had integrated my countertransference disclosure. These vignettes will be followed by a summary analysis of what transpired dynamically in all of them.

CASE EXAMPLES

A Therapist's Resistance to a Client's Erotic Transference

Dr. A., who had received his doctorate in clinical social work, was an experienced practitioner in his early forties, married with one child, and a director of a large social service department in an industrial setting. He impressed me from the very beginning of our supervisory contact as a very skilled clinician, sharp diagnostician, and excellent theoretician, who was very dedicated to his clients and achieved good results in his work with them. He was very eager to learn and seemed to enjoy his work with me as he enjoyed his own private practice. I had been seeing Dr. A. on a weekly basis for about three years, working with him on a variety of case situations, when he presented a client who did not seem to be making any progress. The client, Beverly, was a single woman in her early thirties whom Dr. A. described as "bright, attractive, and very successful in her work as a publicist." What brought Beverly into therapy was her inability to sustain a relationship with a man. By the time she started treatment with Dr. A. (which was several months before he discussed the case with me), she was moderately depressed, had vague psychosomatic complaints, and her "self-esteem was going downhill."

When Dr. A. initially discussed Beverly with me, he pointed out that at the beginning of treatment, Beverly seemed to look forward to her sessions and enjoyed Dr. A.'s accepting attitude and interested listening. This helped her feel less depressed and more hopeful. She found herself to be less critical of men, and, though she did not sustain relationships with them, her interactions with them seemed smoother. Despite Beverly's initial progress, Dr. A. pointed out that lately they seemed to be going in circles. When I asked him to describe the circles, Dr. A. talked about Beverly's flirtatious attitude, which consisted of her giving him all kinds of compliments about his appearance and humane demeanor. When I wondered how Dr. A. felt about Beverly's flattering comments and what he did about them, he became visibly embarrassed and then suggested that Beverly was idealizing him and that this was a transference resistance.

As I listened to Dr. A.'s description of his interaction with Beverly, it became quite clear that the client was becoming very enamored of her therapist but that Dr. A. was subtly rejecting her approaches. This seemed even more evident when I learned that Dr. A. was making genetic interpretations, trying to show Beverly that she was behaving like a young girl looking for a doting father. Dr. A., who usually welcomed my observations on his clients' transference reactions and his countertransference responses, did not relate too well to my suggestion that Beverly was falling in love with him and that it was making him a bit uncomfortable. Rather, he suggested that he needed some help in formulating an interpretation to deal with her transference resistance.

As I reflected on my interaction with Dr. A., I began to see a parallel process developing. Like Beverly, I was saying to Dr. A., "Take note of me, I've got something to offer you," and Dr. A. was politely rejecting both of us. Having studied parallel processes previously with Dr. A., I thought he would be receptive to my statement that both Beverly and I were trying to get closer to him but we weren't being very successful. Instead, he changed the subject and, like the therapy he was conducting, he and I seemed to be going around in circles. After about four to five weeks of trying in vain to help Dr. A. empathize more with Beverly's longings and show him how to make it safer for her to feel her loving and sexual feelings toward him, I decided to share with Dr. A. my countertransference reactions toward him and Beverly. What I was feeling was very sorry for Beverly who was being pushed away. I was also strongly identified with Beverly because I, too, was feeling pushed away by Dr. A. In addition I felt frustrated with Dr. A. because he was not responding lovingly to a woman who wanted to love him. I said to him, "You remind me of a time when I was at a college dance. I was watching a good friend of mine dancing with a girl who was very interested in him. My friend kept dancing far apart from the girl and I wanted him to hug and kiss her instead. I felt like yelling to my friend, 'Why the hell are you treating a woman who wants you that way? Make it better for her and for yourself. Dance closer, God damn it!'"

When Dr. A. listened to my story, he responded with a loud giggle. After the giggling subsided, he said, "Herb, I'm really flattered and feel good that I remind you of a friend of yours. So I feel I'm your friend. I also feel that you have my best interest at heart—you want me to enjoy myself with a woman! Thank you!" In the next supervisory session, Dr. A. came in very enthusiastically. Before sitting down, he said, "It really worked. As soon as Beverly came into my office she said, 'You look different. I think you like me today and so I like you.'" Dr. A. went on to say, "This is just what transpired with us during the last supervisory setting—we both felt closer to each other." When Beverly saw that Dr. A. was more receptive to her loving feelings, she could share some of her sexual fantasies toward him. This helped Dr. A. and Beverly eventually get in touch with a repetition compulsion of hers: seeking out rejecting men like her father, trying to seduce them at first, and then rejecting them before they could reject her. This understanding eventually helped Beverly to form a more sustained relationship with one man.

The Therapist Has Difficulty Beginning Where the Client Is

Ms. C. sought me out for supervision just a few months after beginning her own private practice. She was a single woman in her early thirties employed in a mental health center for about five years as both a practitioner and field work instructor for social work students. In my initial conferences with Ms. C., I experienced her as very outgoing, eager to learn, and possessed of a wealth of warm feelings toward her clients. One of Ms. C.'s major concerns when she started supervision with me was that her clients were leaving her prematurely and she couldn't figure out why. Furthermore, losing clients hardly ever occurred when she worked in the mental health center. In addition, she was able to help her students keep their clients in treatment almost all of the time.

Ms. C. and I agreed that perhaps we would be able to learn what might be causing her clients to leave treatment prematurely if we reviewed together some of her current private cases. As Ms. C. discussed her clients with me, it became quite clear that she was much too active with them. She asked them loads of questions, made many interpretations, and offered them a great deal of reassurance. As I was feeling some annoyance with her, my initial reaction to her presentations (which I kept to myself), was, "She's not giving her clients time or room to speak. How can I get her to calm down and be quieter?" I shared with Ms. C. my impression that she was very active with her clients and wondered if this was her customary way of relating to them at the agency. After seriously thinking about my question she said, "You know, I'm quieter at the center and listen more." Reflecting further on the issue, Ms. C. was able to recognize with just a little help from me that because she was new in private practice and wanted to succeed, she had to work harder for her money or her clients would leave.

Although I thought our discussion would temper Ms. C.'s overactivity with her clients, I was dead wrong! Apparently her anxiety had not abated and she was still unable to listen to them. In two or three instances they even implied this themselves. As I began to study my countertransference reactions to Ms. C. further, I realized that I was becoming quite frustrated and impatient with her. In addition I realized that I was becoming too active with her. I tried to get her to just listen but to no avail. I tried to discuss her anxiety about being in private practice and though she thought our discussions were illuminating, they got us nowhere. I even lent her some literature but that did not help either.

When my teaching role was clearly not working, I decided to share some of my countertransference reactions directly with Ms. C. I told her, "I'm feeling very inept with you. I'm working hard to help you relax and it's not helping you. What's wrong with me?" To this Ms. C. said with a twinkle in her eye, "I'm reassured that you can consider yourself a failure. I think I've been working very hard with my clients so that I won't fail with them. Maybe if I could accept the fact that failing isn't so bad, I'd relax more with my clients." Ms. C.'s remarks made me feel a lot warmer and closer to her. As a result I was then able to share with her some of my initial experiences in the army where I was a young social work officer, eager to succeed, but worried that I would not. I recalled one time when a G.I. came to the mental hygiene clinic suffering from a severe migraine headache. Instead of letting him talk, I took his history. As a result, his headache got worse. Ms. C. laughed heartily at my story and said, "I've got to be less serious in the interviews with my clients."

Ms. C.'s overactivity with her clients clearly induced in me a wish to be overactive with her. When I shared the feelings of ineptness that helped create my overactivity with her, Ms. C. could be more relaxed with me and then with her clients. Not to our surprise, the clients we had been discussing remained in treatment.

A Marriage Counselor Takes Sides

Mr. D., a married man in his late forties with two children, was in full-time private practice for about ten years, specializing in marriage counseling. He had been in supervision about two years, discussing his couple counseling with much animation, confidence, and pleasure. Accomplished in his specialty, he published articles in his field of practice and was well regarded by his colleagues. I felt close to him and enjoyed working with him. Until we began working with the case under discussion, our supervisory work had moved positively and we both felt we were growing professionally from it.

During his third year of supervision, Mr. D. wanted to spend some time on a case that was going nowhere. Eric and Flora had been seeing Mr. D. for close to a year. Flora was feeling very hostile and disappointed with Eric because he hardly ever wanted to have sex, was always distant from her, and made her feel unappreciated. Eric, on the other hand, felt nagged, pressured, and misunderstood. Mr. D. felt that no matter what he did in the sessions, the couple kept bickering and became even more alienated from each other. As I listened to Mr. D.'s descriptions of his sessions with Eric and Flora, it became quite clear that almost every time Flora talked, Mr. D. would emerge as very supportive and empathetic, but almost every time Eric participated, Mr. D. said nothing. When I shared my observation with Mr. D., he responded, "The guy doesn't have much to offer, so I don't have much to support." I suggested that this was just what Flora was feeling, so, in effect, he, Mr. D., was more identified with Flora and less with Eric.

Although Mr. D. could acknowledge his countertransference reactions toward Flora and Eric—sympathetic toward Flora and mildly contemptuous toward Eric—it did not alter his way of relating to them. He continued to favor Flora and the marriage kept floundering. Furthermore, suggestions on my part that Flora unconsciously wanted a withdrawn man and that Eric felt very vulnerable did not modify Mr. D.'s biased treatment. In sharing my countertransference with Mr. D. I said, "You know, as I work with you on this case, I feel very different from the way I do with other marital situations that we've discussed. In virtually every other one, I feel included in the system. In this one, I feel ignored, as if I'm a bump on a log. There's something going on for both of us because you, too, have not been satisfied with the movement in this case."

After a long silence, Mr. D. told me that one word I used

brought tears to his eyes. "That is the word 'ignored'," he said with much emotion. Without prompting, he shared with me how very ignored he had felt as a child in his own family. Frequently, he felt like a scapegoat in that he experienced his parents and brother as always ganging up on him. After I commented, "You've had it rough," Mr. D. responded, "I guess I've been wanting to get you and Flora to gang up with me against Eric. Eric kind of reminds me of my older brother, and I'd like to give him a taste of his own medicine. Without realizing it, I'm doing to Eric what was done to me in my own family. I'm identifying with the aggressor."

When Mr. D. could see that he was unconsciously arranging to treat Eric the way he was treated in his own family, he began to listen to him more, empathize with him more, and try to show him that he understood what an outsider feels like. This modified attitude on Mr. D.'s part helped the marital therapy move forward a great deal and helped Eric and Flora to communicate with each other in a more mature manner. Their sex life improved and their emotional distance from each other diminished tremendously.

A Fee Problem Goes Unaddressed

Dr. G., a divorced woman in her fifties, was in full-time private practice, and had been in supervision with me for close to a year. Although bright, engaging, and very committed to her clients, Dr. G. appeared overinvolved in their lives. She tended to give advice when it was not asked for, intervened in their environments when the clients might have been able to use their own resources, and offered a great deal of reassurance that did not always seem indicated. A case that Dr. G. wanted to discuss with me in more breadth and depth involved a client, Mr. H., who Dr. G. felt was a psychopath. Mr. H., an accountant, cheated his clients, was unfaithful to his wife, neglected his children, and gossiped about his friends.

He started treatment with Dr. G. about two years prior to her discussion of the case with me, after his physician told him that his psychosomatic problems were caused by stress.

As I listened to Dr. G.'s description of Mr. H., I was baffled by a number of issues. Although Dr. G. referred to Mr. H. pejoratively as a psychopath, in the treatment she was warm, tender, and what appeared to me as quite indulgent. I was shocked that she let him owe her well over $2,000 and hadn't explored this resistance in the treatment. Despite his obvious rage at his wife, children, and associates, Dr. G. neglected this as well. When I asked her why she let a big debt accumulate, she told me that her client was broke but that she wanted to help him clear up his debt and this was the only way she knew how to do it. I found Dr. G.'s responses to my other queries quite similar. "The poor guy needs support," "he's never been given to," "I feel sorry for him" were some of them.

Inasmuch as I felt that Dr. G.'s treatment of Mr. H. would not get off the ground until she was firmer with him and had him explore his mistreatment of her, I shared this conviction with Dr. G. and said, firmly, "He's taking advantage of you, too. Find out why he's not paying you!" When Dr. G. essentially evaded my suggestion, I felt she was behaving with me the same way her client was behaving with her, and not paying attention to my need to be listened to. I then said, "Just as Mr. H. owes you money and should pay you, I think you might consider taking my suggestion seriously," trying to demonstrate to Dr. G. how to be firm. However, Dr. G. responded by saying that I was being too rough on her and that I wanted her to be too rough on her client. When I became aware that all my interventions with Dr. G. were not helpful to her or to her client, I decided to share some of my countertransference reactions with her. As already implied, I had a load of intense feelings. I was contemptuous of and angry at Mr. H. for exploiting Dr. G. I was irritated with Dr. G. for letting herself be so mistreated. I speculated that just as Dr. G. and Mr. H. were ignoring the fee problem, Dr. G. and I must not be paying attention to something in our relationship because we weren't getting anywhere in our communication.

It seemed to me that the best way to try to reach Dr. G. was to demonstrate the parallel process that I thought was occurring. Therefore, I said, "Just as you and Mr. H. seem to be ignoring the fee and going on with your work but not getting very far, you and I must be ignoring something in our relationship because we are not getting very far either!" As if she had been waiting to tell me for a long time, Dr. G. said, "Yes, we're ignoring the fact that I want to be your friend and colleague and you treat me as if I'm just one of your supervisees. You could be a lot warmer to me, ask me out for lunch occasionally, take a walk with me. What's wrong with you?"

As I reflected on Dr. G.'s question about what was wrong with me, I came up with the following answer which I then shared with her. "What's wrong with me is that I haven't been the kind of guy you've wanted me to be. For a year now you've wanted a friendship with me and I've been seeing you only in my office. I didn't realize how much I've been frustrating you!" Dr. G. responded with enormous indignation: "I think your response is full of coldness and hostility. There's no reason why we can't be buddies on the outside and colleagues on the inside. You are much too formal!"

My sharing of my countertransference with Dr. G. was initially more helpful to me than it was to her. By looking at what we were not facing in our work, I not only learned that I was deflecting Dr. G.'s wishes to be a friend, but I saw what I was not attending to in the supervision. Dr. G. wanted me to treat her the way she was treating Mr. H. and instead I was the controlled professional who did not gratify her yearnings for contact and did not discuss this important issue with her.

Once I became sensitized to the fact that Dr. G. wanted me to indulge her the way she was indulging Mr. H., I could become more relaxed and therefore more of an enabler. Instead of being irritated with her for not following my supervisory suggestions, I could empathize with her personal loneliness and help her see that she was trying to make her supervisor and her client into boyfriends. Although Dr. G. never entirely gave up her quest to use her professional relationships for personal gain, in time she could be more limiting and more confronting with Mr. H. and with other clients. As she could slowly adapt to my limit-setting (which became warmer and less mechanical), she could eventually set limits for Mr. H. and help him pay up his fee. Concomitant with his paying his debt, Mr. H. because more considerate of his family, clients, and friends.

DISCUSSION OF CASES

In attempting to assess dynamically the four vignettes just presented, it would appear that the material affirms several traditional principles of social work supervision and also generates a few hypotheses that may enable social work supervisors to become more sensitive and competent enablers.

Just as every well-motivated client in psychotherapy resists learning about herself, the supervisee who wants to learn more about himself also needs to protect himself from facing vulnerabilities and resists supervision. Furthermore, similar to the patient in psychotherapy who unconsciously arranges to distort the therapist, the supervisee usually has a wide range of transference reactions toward the supervisor. Some of these can accelerate learning while others can inhibit it.

None of the four supervisees discussed were required to have supervision. Similar to voluntary patients who spend time and money to improve themselves, but also concomitantly have to avoid danger, the supervisees under discussion all resisted my teaching at various points. Dr. A. did not want to face his client's erotic transference, Ms. C. did not want to confront her therapeutic overactivity, Mr. D. was not eager to face the reasons he was biased in the marital counseling, and Dr. G. resisted confronting her indulgence of her client.

In all of the four cases the parallel process became evident in that the transference–countertransference interaction that took place in the therapy was recapitulated in the transference–countertransference interaction between me and my supervisees. Dr. A. and I could not easily communicate about love and sex and this was true in his work with Beverly. Ms. C. and I were not able to listen carefully to each other, and this was clearly happening with Ms. C. and her clients. I felt ignored by Mr. D., and this is what he was doing with Eric. Dr. G. wanted me to indulge her as she was indulging her patient, but this was a secret in the supervision, as it was in the therapy she was conducting. When I observed that my supervisees did not respond positively to my teaching or my clarifications and interpretations of the parallel process, I decided to disclose some of my countertransference reactions to them. In all four cases, the tension between us then diminished, the supervisory alliance became stronger, and the therapeutic impasse moved toward resolution. Why did this happen?

I believe that just as in psychotherapy, when the therapist abdicates his traditional role of interpreter and expert and shares his vulnerabilities, the therapeutic impasse moves toward resolution (Strean 1999), so, too, in supervision. Dr. A. began to see me more as a colleague and an equal rather than as a judge and a critic. Ms. C., when she could experience me as fallible and capable of making mistakes, was able to allow herself to feel fallible with her clients and therefore became more relaxed in the treatment situation. Dr. D. could acknowledge his unconscious rejection of Eric when I discussed my feelings of being rejected. Dr. G. could face her wishes to indulge her client when I could more directly discuss my feelings about indulging her.

The supervisor's disclosure of her countertransference tends to make her appear as much less authoritarian, more egalitarian, less of a wise expert and more of an authentic human being. This humane attitude of the supervisor helps reduce the supervisee's self-consciousness and need to appear omniscient. As the supervisor relinquishes some of her grandiose wishes to be a know-it-all, the supervisee tends to do the same. A more relaxed therapist then makes for a more relaxed client and the therapeutic alliance is strengthened. What was most impressive about the cases under review is that the supervisor's disclosing of the countertransference activated a different treatment interaction from the one that contributed to the therapeutic impasse. From going around in circles, Dr. A. and Beverly could more honestly discuss love and sex. Ms. C. could become a better listener and thus her clients began to stay in treatment. Mr. D. became less hostile and Eric and Flora improved their marital interaction. Dr. G. became less indulgent and Mr. H. evolved into a more decent human being.

As my supervisees observed that I was taking some initiative in disclosing my feelings of anger, hurt, rejection, and so forth, they felt a freedom to identify with me and do the same. And, when I did not reveal very much about myself, they also tended to be withholding. In effect, the supervisor was experienced in all four cases as a role model who set the tone of the interaction. If I was revealing, the supervisee was more inclined to be revealing. And when the supervisee felt less anxiety about revealing himself, he invariably made it safer for his client to face herself. One of the positive effects of disclosing the supervisor's countertransference is that it tends to clarify the supervisee's transference toward her. This was particularly true in the case of Dr. G., who was harboring negative feelings toward me of which I was unaware, and dependent and sexual yearnings, which I tended to deflect.

In reviewing my work with the supervisees under study, I feel quite certain that if I had not disclosed my countertransference reactions, the therapeutic impasses would not have been resolved. The supervisor's disclosure of her countertransference strengthens the supervisory alliance, which in turn strengthens the therapeutic alliance.

CONCLUSION

It is common in most supervisory relationships for the supervisee to resist confronting certain dynamic issues in his client and in himself. These issues usually become expressed in the transference–countertransference interaction between the supervisee and his supervisor. Mutual examination of this supervisory interaction often clarifies what is transpiring in the therapeutic relationship. When mutual examination bogs down, the supervisor's disclosure of her countertransference appears to strengthen the supervisory alliance. This in turn enables the therapist to strengthen the therapeutic alliance with his client, which can then help resolve a therapeutic impasse.

It is hoped that further research on the supervisor's disclosure of her countertransference will be conducted. Is such disclosure helpful at times other than during a therapeutic impasse? How helpful is it in supervisory groups or seminars? When supervisors convene to enhance their skills, would mutual sharing of their countertransference reactions to their supervisees improve their supervisory work? Finally, are there any negative effects of the supervisor disclosing her countertransference responses?

REFERENCES

Abend, S. (1982). Serious illness in the analyst: countertransference considerations. *Journal of the American Psychoanalytic Association* 30:365–379.

——— (1989). Countertransference and psychoanalytic technique. *Psychoanalytic Quarterly* 58:374–396.

Arlow, J. (1963). The supervisory situation. *Journal of the American Psychoanalytic Association* 11:576–594.

Balint, M. (1948). On the psychoanalytic training system. *International Journal of Psycho-Analysis* 29:163–173.

Barchilon, J. (1958). On countertransference cures. *Journal of the American Psychoanalytic Association* 6:222–236.

Bibring, G. (1950). Psychiatry and social work. In *Principles and Techniques in Social Casework*, ed. C. Kasius, pp. 300–313. New York: Family Service Association of America.

Brenner, C. (1985). Countertransference as a compromise formation. *Psychoanalytic Quarterly* 54(2):155–163.

Chessick, R. (1971). *Why Psychotherapists Fail*. New York: Jason Aronson.

Doehrman, M. (1976). Parallel processes in supervision and psychotherapy. *Bulletin of the Menninger Clinic* 40:9–84.

Ekstein, R., and Wallerstein, R. (1972). *The Teaching and Learning of Psychotherapy*. New York: International Universities Press.

Feldman, Y. (1950). The teaching aspect of casework supervision. In *Principles of Techniques in Social Casework*, ed. C. Kasius, pp. 222–232. New York: Family Service Association of America.

Fine, R. (1982). *The Healing of the Mind*, 2nd edition. New York: Free Press.

Fleming, J., and Benedek, T. (1966). *Psychoanalytic Supervision*. New York: Grune & Stratton.

Freud, S. (1910). The future prospects of psycho-analytic therapy. *Standard Edition* 11:141–151.

——— (1912). The dynamics of transference. *Standard Edition*. 12:99–108.

——— (1915). Observations on transference-love. *Standard Edition* 12:159–173.

——— (1919). Lines of advance in psychoanalytic therapy. *Standard Edition* 17:159–168.

——— (1926). Inhibitions, symptoms and anxiety. *Standard Edition* 20:77–175.

Glover, E. (1952). Research methods in psychoanalysis. *International Journal of Psycho-Analysis* 33:403–409.

Greenson, R. (1967). *The Technique and Practice of Psychoanalysis*. New York: International Universities Press.

Heimann, P. (1950). On countertransference. *International Journal of Psycho-Analysis* 31:81–84.

Issacharoff, A. (1984). Countertransference in supervision: therapeutic consequences for the supervisee. In *Critical Perspectives on the Supervision of Psychoanalysis and Psychotherapy*, ed. L. Caligor, P. M. Bromberg, and J. D. Meltzer, pp. 89–105. New York: Plenum.

Jacobs, T. (1986). On countertransference enactments. *Journal of the American Psychoanalytic Association* 43:289–307.

Lane, R. (1990). *Psychoanalytic Approaches to Supervision*. New York: Brunner/Mazel.

Langs, R. (1979). *The Supervisory Experience*. New York: Jason Aronson.

Lesser, R. (1984). Supervision: illustrations, anxieties, and questions. In *Clinical Perspectives on the Supervision of Psychoanalysis and Psychotherapy*, ed. L. Caligor, P. M. Bromberg, and J. D. Meltzer, pp. 143–152. New York: Plenum.

Marshall, R. (1997). The interactional triad in supervision. In *Psychodynamic Supervision*, ed. M. Rock, pp. 77–106. Northvale, NJ: Jason Aronson.

Reich, A. (1951). On countertransference. In *Psychoanalytic Contributions*, ed. A. Reich, pp. 136–154. New York: International Universities Press.

Richmond, M. (1917). *Social Diagnosis*. New York: Russell Sage Foundation.

Rock, M. (1997). *Psychodynamic Supervision*. Northvale, NJ: Jason Aronson.

Sandler, J. (1976). Countertransference and role responsiveness. *International Review of Psycho-Analysis* 3:43–48.

Schlesinger, H. (1981). General principles of psychoanalytic

supervision. In *Becoming a Psychoanalyst*, ed. R. Wallerstein, pp. 29–38. New York: International Universities
Press.

Searles, H. (1955). The informational value of the supervisor's
emotional experience. In *Collected Papers on Schizophrenia and Related Subjects*, ed. H. Searles, pp. 157–176.
New York: International Universities Press, 1965.

——— (1962). Problems of psychoanalytic supervision. In
Collected Papers on Schizophrenia, ed. H. Searles, pp.
584–604. New York: International Universities Press,
1965.

Strean, H. (1986). *Behind the Couch*. New York: Wiley.

——— (1988). Colluding illusions among analytic candidates,
their supervisors, and their patients: a major factor in
some treatment impasses. *Psychoanalytic Psychology* 8:
403–414.

——— (1999). Resolving some therapeutic impasses by disclosing countertransference. *Clinical Social Work Journal*
27:123–140.

Teitelbaum, S. (1990). Supertransference: the role of the
supervisor's blind spots. *Psychoanalytic Psychology* 7(2):
243–258.

Williams, M. (1965). *Supervision: New Patterns and Processes*.
New York: Free Association Press.

Wolman, B. (1972). *Success and Failure in Psychoanalysis and
Psychotherapy*. New York: Macmillan.

Discussion:
The Supervisee's Response
to the Supervisor's
Self-Disclosure

Gildo Consolini

Dr. Herbert Strean makes an important contribution to the clinical social work literature by extending his discussion of self-disclosure of countertransference to the use of such disclosure in clinical supervision. As he did in his paper on the use of such disclosure in psychotherapeutic treatment, Strean (1999) demonstrates with his case illustrations how the discussion of countertransferential responses enables the therapist to resolve certain treatment impasses. Just as the disclosure of the therapist's emotional reactions to his patient can lead to a strengthening of the therapeutic alliance, the disclosure of the supervisor's emotional reactions to her supervisee can strengthen the supervisory alliance. In treatment, the patient becomes more receptive to the interpretive activity of the therapist, which is necessary to resolve a treatment impasse. In supervision, the supervisee becomes more willing and able to use what the supervisor can teach him about psychoanalytic theory and technique to resolve an impasse that has developed between the supervisee and the patient.

I am very pleased to have this opportunity to respond to Dr. Strean's paper. I hope that I can add something to what he has said by describing some of my own supervisory experiences. Specifically, I will compare my response to supervision in which countertransference disclosure was for the most part avoided to my response in supervision when such disclosure was used to address treatment impasses. However, I would first like to comment about two of the issues Strean raises in his review of the literature on supervision: the complexity of the contemporary supervisory role and the supervisor's theoretical and technical knowledge base.

THE EVOLUTION OF THE SUPERVISORY ROLE SET

As Dr. Strean describes, for many years the social work supervisor's function was essentially administrative until the expectation developed by the 1960s that the supervisor also assume a teaching function. As the use of psychoanalytic concepts became widespread in mental health practice, supervision became a means of teaching these concepts to therapists, and the supervisor used his analytic knowledge to develop an assessment of the learning needs of the supervisee. Currently, the shift from a one-person to a two-person psychology in treatment is reflected in a corresponding shift in the conceptualization of how supervision may be conducted. With this shift comes a risk that some of the complexity that Strean recognizes in his conceptualization of the supervisory process will be lost sight of.

The expectation that the supervisor will now look more carefully at what transpires interpersonally and intersubjectively in supervision and respond effectively to these psychodynamic aspects of this work does not eliminate the other functions the supervisor is expected to fulfill. That is, the supervisor continues to need to teach theory and technique to virtually every supervisee, often must make an evaluation of the supervisee's progress or lack thereof, and may be required to provide administrative as well as clinical supervision of the therapist. Although Strean endorses the contemporary shift to a two-person psychology, he reminds us that new roles have been added to the role set of the supervisor without relinquishment of any of the traditional supervisory functions.

In a recent exploration of the implications of contemporary relational perspectives for field instruction in social work, Ganzer and Orenstein (1999) use case vignettes to illustrate how relational theory enriches the understanding of the relationship between field instructor and student and makes their collaboration more effective. They do an excellent job of relocating parallel process in a larger relational matrix by demonstrating the role of the supervisor's dynamics in the development of learning impasses that parallel treatment impasses. However, while the use of a relational approach to alter the hierarchical aspects of the relationship between supervisor and supervisee may encourage the supervisee to take more initiative in his learning, it may also serve to deny some of the realities of the relationship. Aron (1996) states that while the analyst wishes to promote mutuality in the treatment relationship, there is an inevitable asymmetry because of the inherent differences in the patient's and analyst's roles, functions, and responsibilities. To deny in supervision that the supervisor needs to provide information to the supervisee that needs to be retained and used, that an ongoing evaluation of her suitability to do the work is being conducted, and that the supervisor often must ensure that the supervisee attends to administrative aspects of her practice, would ultimately hinder the professional development of the therapist.

Itzhaky and Stern (1999) examine the pseudo-parental role of the supervisor to make us aware that supervision of young therapists can slip rather easily into a parent–child mode. They propose a method to prevent transferential and countertransferential feelings that so easily develop between the supervisor and his supervisee from intruding on the supervision. Their support model helps remind the supervisor of the differences between the supervisor–supervisee relationship and the parent–child relationship during stressful periods in the work when it can be compelling to ignore these differences. As Strean indicates, the contemporary supervisor is compelled to transcend the traditional teach-or-treat dilemma by assuming some responsibility for both activities. Traditionally, the supervisor was discouraged from doing more than directing the supervisee back to treatment when a personal issue of the supervisee that was interfering in her clinical work was identified. Many authors have indicated that a good deal of probing is required during supervisory sessions to resolve the issue sufficiently to get the supervisee's work with her patient back on track (e.g., Lane 1990). Itzhaky and Stern (1999) call the supervisor's reluctance to inquire into the emotions of the supervisee that develop during treatment, on the grounds that to do so is abandoning supervision for therapy, a pretext for absolving the supervisor of his responsibility to discuss any emotions that may be hindering treatment.

In addition to the potential risk of using relational theory to deny the reality of the hierarchical aspects of the supervisory relationship, there is also the risk of denying the reality of other differences in the effort to promote mutuality in supervisory work. This denial can cause further difficulty when the supervisor attempts to teach, administer, or oversee practice. More often than not, the supervisor is much more established and accomplished professionally, significantly older than the supervisee, and has much more clinical knowledge and experience. Thus, not only does the supervisor have a responsibility to teach, he is also likely to have a great deal to offer as a mentor. As Billow (1999) suggests, the supervisor as well as the supervisee may have rather strong and largely unexamined feelings of entitlement concerning what is being offered and not being offered to the supervisee as well as how the supervisee responds to these offerings and non-offerings. His case examples illustrate the use of an intersubjective approach to identify such expressions in both participants in the supervisory relationship.

GAPS IN KNOWLEDGE AND DELAYS IN THE USE OF KNOWLEDGE

Rock (1997) comments that, despite the fact that supervision is central to training and professional development in all of the mental health disciplines, "little attention has been devoted to discussions of the nature of the process and the factors which contribute to its effectiveness or ineffectiveness" (p. 3). The shift in psychoanalytic theory from the "drive/structure" to the "relational/structure" model of development (Greenberg and Mitchell 1983) provides those who are writing currently with a better conceptual framework for such discussions. As Strean makes clear, it has become commonplace for authors to recognize the bidirectionality of the therapeutic process and to promote mutuality in the treatment relationship.

Rock (1997) points out that although changes in the psychoanalytic theory of supervision have paralleled paradigmatic shifts in psychoanalytic theory, these changes have occurred at a slower rate. A very basic but important aspect of this contribution by Strean to the literature on supervision is his timely application of knowledge gained from the recent study of psychotherapeutic technique to supervision. As Strean indicates, although Searles observed more than forty years ago that the disclosure of the inner experience of the supervisor could have great value, it is only recently that the supervisor's self-disclosure is getting the attention in the literature it deserves.

Within a year of his paper on countertransference disclosure in treatment (1999), Strean followed with this paper on the use of such disclosure in supervision. Perhaps there will be less delay from now on in the transmission of knowledge from one activity to the next, as indicated also by Billow's recent (1999) contribution. In the same paper Billow examines how entitlement is expressed by the two participants in supervision as well as in treatment and describes an intersubjective approach to its uncovering and management.

The general reluctance to use what has been learned from the treatment process to understand the supervisory process seems to be lessening as the supervisor, to use Strean's words, "comes out of the closet" to his supervisee. As Strean also indicates in his review, Fleming and Benedek (1966) contributed the concept of the "learning alliance" in supervision some time ago, a notion that parallels Greenson's "therapeutic alliance" (1967). It seems those now writing are better prepared to understand the basis for constructive activity that strengthens the alliance in supervision as a result of the theoretical and technical developments Strean refers to in his paper.

One can only imagine how much better supervision could have been for many if theorists had been more willing and better able to apply what has been learned about therapeutic action to supervision. Strean also makes reference in his paper to a book about psychoanalytic approaches to supervision edited by Lane (1990). In one of the papers in this book, Lane and Hull do an excellent job of applying Kris's (1956) classic conceptualization, from an ego psychological perspective, of what happens when treatment is working to understand the "good hour" in supervision. Here again, it took many years for someone to realize the value of such a concept in supervision and to write about it.

With his case illustrations, Strean offers us an additional basis for the development of the supervisory alliance that builds upon an intersubjective approach to clinical work. Stolorow and Atwood (1992) claim that the therapeutic alliance is established in treatment as a result of the commitment on the part of the analyst to investigate dysfunction in the analytic relationship from within the perspective of the patient's own subjective reality. This investigation creates the therapeutic context for the uncovering of the patient's unconscious organizing principles, making therapeutic transformation possible. Strean shows that something very similar can happen in supervision when the supervisor and supervisee can openly discuss their emotional reactions to each other at apparent points of impasse.

TWENTY YEARS OF SUPERVISION: SOME OBSERVATIONS

After more than twenty years of being supervised, nearly twenty years of supervising others, and learning throughout these years about the experiences of other supervisees and supervisors, I can safely say that dissatisfaction with the supervisory process and situation is common. That is not to say that practitioners do not often benefit a great deal from both the experience of being supervised and supervising others—I know that I certainly have. However, it seems that certain common problems that develop between the participants in supervision are addressed more effectively when the supervisor is more active in initiating a discussion of transferential and countertransferential feelings. The selective disclosure by the supervisor of his own inner experience is an especially important aspect of such a process.

Early in my social work career, I had a disturbing experience with a supervisor at the very beginning of our relationship that decisively affected, for the worse, the remainder of our work together. After working in a medical setting for two months with minimal supervision, I was scheduled to meet with my new supervisor for the first time. I was very anxious about this meeting, eager to prove myself. I believed I was well regarded by the medical staff, had done rather well in her absence, and hoped she would appreciate this. Also, I was to be the first of eight supervisees with whom she would be meeting, which made me feel special (a feeling that resonated from my experience as the eldest of six children). What she did was far from terrible; however, I was so hurt and angry that it made it very hard for me to listen to anything she said for the rest of the year.

She kept me waiting for almost two hours before we met. It is hard to recall how long the wait actually was because it seemed more like days than like hours, and more importantly, I was determined to not allow myself to be emotionally affected. I am sure there was a good reason for her delay. When we did begin, she may have explained or apologized about the delay—I do not remember one way or the other. Furthermore, she did not seem very impressed at all when I told her about my work with my patients. Since my walls were up, it is likely that she did not realize how upset I was. In any case, my perception was that I was being regarded as a very insignificant person. I acted out my feelings toward her throughout our year together by challenging virtually every-thing she said in her teaching role. As I had done as an adolescent, if it seemed I would not get enough attention by doing things as I had been taught I would become opposi-tional. Since she favored a psychoanalytic approach in most cases, I insisted instead on using behavior modification or a family systems approach with my clients. When she encour-aged me to help my clients find resources within themselves to solve their problems, I insisted instead that I needed to act on their behalf and intervene in their environment.

Perhaps things would have gone better if we had been able to discuss what had happened when we first got together.

For my part, I believed our supervisory conference was simply not the place for me to express what I was feeling about anybody, let alone my supervisor. Like so many individuals who have difficulty dealing with those in authority, I have benefited greatly whenever an authority figure has encouraged me to find a constructive way to express my feelings, particularly about my relationship with him or her.

I have been fortunate to have had very positive experiences with the supervision I received during my analytic training. I learned a great deal from each of my three talented supervisors, a woman and two men. However, a recurrent difficulty I had with each was not uncovered until I began working with Dr. Strean, about three years following the completion of my training. I am inclined to think that, specifically, his willingness to share his feelings with me, along with his general skill in addressing the parallel process, made this possible. In addition to working with Herb on an individual basis, I also participated in a group for supervisors that he led.

Both with me individually and in his group, Herb actively encouraged the sharing of associations to the material from supervisory sessions that was presented. This clarified the parallel process time and again. He also was very generous in his praise. Coltart (1996), I think rather beautifully, indicates the value of praise in her discussion of postgraduate supervision.

> I do believe that in supervision, in therapy, and indeed in our ordinary lives, we sometimes need to remind ourselves that we can genuinely enhance the life of someone else if we put into words a considered, experienced, and positive opinion of that person rather than just thinking it. The grudging fears, often encountered in psychoanalysts, that we shall have some grim negative influence by this sort of behavior, represent one of the less-attractive aspects

of psychoanalysis and are, I think, rooted in a primitive, Calvinistic sort of morality approaching superstition, rather than in rational thought or even human experience. [pp. 149–150]

I was certainly enjoying the praise I was receiving from Herb, among other aspects of my work with him.

Not long after I began working with Herb, I had a dream in which I was attempting to speak with him about a case. In the dream, I was looking forward to doing so when I realized, as I opened my notebook, that I had nothing written in it. The feeling of panic was so strong that I woke up. As I had done with other supervisors, however, I did not tell Herb about the dream for some time. I continued to believe that such a dream was something to be dealt with through one's self-analysis rather than through supervision.

What eventually led me to change my mind about this was Herb's sharing some of his emotional reactions to my patients, to me, and to what my patients and I were attempting to do with each other when therapeutic impasses developed. It became clear that I was much more concerned with impressing him than I needed to be. This made it easier for me to bring in something I did my best to avoid bringing in to other supervisors I had had—the mistakes I made over and over again. Not that my supervisors were unaware of these mistakes, at least not those who were knowledgeable enough to understand my defenses. The problem was that pointing them out had a limited effect. The timing was often not right for dealing with my countertransferential feelings in my special analysis and it did not seem appropriate to discuss these feelings in depth during supervision. I did my best to hide my difficulties. Thus, if I repeatedly failed to make a certain interpretation with a particular patient, I stopped bringing his material into supervision. I also stopped bringing that kind of patient up at all. Eventually, I found myself talking only about my least disturbed patients, those with whom working classically was the least problematic.

If the overall unconscious goal of supervision becomes impressing your supervisor or avoiding his criticism, one will have great difficulty using one's supervisor's help to find effective ways of working analytically with narcissistically vulnerable and borderline patients. With such patients, one can easily perceive oneself to be a poorly functioning analytic practitioner. At least this was my experience. It was not until I became comfortable enough to bring in those cases in which the work was proceeding the least smoothly, when I could admit feeling helpless or defeated, or that I was less than fond of the patient, that I began to make real headway with these individuals.

When someone as seasoned, talented, and optimistic as Herb is able to admit such feelings it makes it much easier to tolerate them within oneself. Again, that was my experience. Furthermore, I have found in my supervision of others that this also holds true. My openness with my supervisees has consistently facilitated a much more honest look at someone else's practice than would be possible if my anonymity induced my supervisees to cover up their difficulties and disturbing emotional reactions to patients in an attempt to earn my praise or avoid my criticism.

CONCLUSION

What Maroda (1995) says about analytic treatment applies as well to analytic supervision. "Show some emotion!" In his paper, Herbert Strean has done a wonderful job of showing us how well this can work. My experience working with him in supervision and using what he has taught me about the use of self-disclosure in my supervision of others corroborates his point of view.

REFERENCES

Aron, L. (1996). *A Meeting of Minds: Mutuality in Psychoanalysis*. Hillsdale, NJ: Analytic Press.

Billow, R. (1999). An intersubjective approach to entitlement. *Psychoanalytic Quarterly* 68:441–461.

Coltart, N. (1996). And now for something completely different: postgraduate supervision. In *Psychodynamic Supervision: Perspectives of the Supervisor and the Supervisee*, ed. M. Rock, pp. 133–155. Northvale, NJ: Jason Aronson, 1997.

Fleming, J., and Benedek, T. (1966). *Psychoanalytic Supervision*. New York: Grune & Stratton.

Ganzer, C., and Orenstein, E. (1999). Beyond parallel process: relational perspectives on field instruction. *Clinical Social Work Journal* 27:231–246.

Greenberg, J., and Mitchell, S. (1983). *Object Relations in Psychoanalytic Theory*. Cambridge, MA: Harvard University Press.

Greenson, R. (1967). *The Technique and Practice of Psychoanalysis*. New York: International Universities Press.

Itzhaky, H., and Stern, L. (1999). The take over of parent–child dynamics in a supervisory relationship: identifying the role transformation. *Clinical Social Work Journal* 27:247–258.

Kris, E. (1956). Some vicissitudes of insight in psychoanalysis. *International Journal of Psycho-Analysis* 37:445–455.

Lane, R. (1990). *Psychoanalytic Approaches to Supervision*. New York: Brunner/Mazel.

Maroda, K. (1995). *Show some emotion: completing the cycle of affective communication*. Paper presented at meeting of the Division of Psychoanalysis (39), American Psychological Association, Santa Monica, CA, April.

Rock, M. (1997). *Psychodynamic Supervision: Perspectives of the Supervisor and the Supervisee*. Northvale, NJ: Jason Aronson.

Stolorow, R., and Atwood, G. (1992). *Contexts of Being: The Intersubjective Foundations of Psychological Life*. Hillsdale, NJ: Analytic Press.

Strean, H. (1999). Resolving some therapeutic impasses by disclosing countertransference. *Clinical Social Work Journal* 27:123–140.

Discussion: Understanding Countertransference as a Liberating Force

Harriet Klein

Supervision in the social work profession is an administrative process that is typically and traditionally utilized in most hospital and social work agencies. While functioning in an administrative role, a social work supervisor can and should integrate a theoretical and clinical process. This permits the supervisor to sharpen the skills of the supervisee while ensuring that the regulations of the hospital or agency are complied with.

Supervising individuals who are in private practice is a different experience. One is not limited by the restrictions and regulations of the hospital or agency. The sole focus is the growth and development of the supervisee as a therapist.

Both, however, have a common thread, which is the relationship. In some respects supervision has many parallels with individual treatment of patients, including the level of intimacy and the many conscious and unconscious issues for both parties involved. Dr. Strean discusses these issues in his paper and brings to light some interesting ideas about the relationship between the supervisor and supervisee. He notes how for many years it was generally believed that when an impasse was presented and discussed in a supervisory relationship the source of the problem was solely the supervisee. The supervisor, supposedly more experienced and better analyzed, was thought to play no role in the impasse in the treatment and would simply show the supervisee how to resolve the matter.

Dr. Strean posits the idea that a more productive supervision involves the supervisor's use of his own countertransference to assist the supervisee in moving the treatment ahead. Here are some case examples of supervisees that demonstrate the countertransference aspects of the supervisory relationship.

> Mr. B. is a man in his mid-thirties. He has a private practice and has been a successful therapist for eight years. He has a number of clients whom we follow and review in supervision. Mr. B. is bright, enthusiastic, and articulate. He evokes a variety of thoughts and feelings in me about the idea of conflict in the supervisory relationship. He would talk about his clients with great frustration, never feeling appreciated enough. He would say, "I feel like I always give and never get." He was overly active in sessions, gave a great deal of advice to his clients, and was not very aware of the effect that his activity and advice-giving had on them. He would talk about his outrage when clients would cancel sessions, call at the last minute, or not call at all. He dwelled on one client who would always call and ask to reschedule or change the time of his session.
>
> We would spend hour after hour in supervision discussing what was going on in his sessions. We would examine the material of the sessions, but he always felt manipulated and put out. We would discuss the dynamics of the sessions, but he didn't quite understand his part in perpetuating these dynamics.
>
> I began to realize that something interesting was taking place in our supervisory relationship. Mr. B.

would endlessly call me to reschedule his hour or to change his weekly time for one reason or another.

I noticed how I was becoming increasingly angry, feeling manipulated and put out myself. I decided to share these feelings with Mr. B. I told him he was doing the same thing with me that his clients were doing with him. He, of course, could not see this. He insisted that his reasons for canceling were legitimate while his clients' cancellations had no justification.

I then realized we were doing the same dance in our sessions. I felt the same angry feelings he felt. It wasn't until I confronted Mr. B. about his wish to be accommodated and his sense of entitlement that he could then interpret this in his sessions with his own clients. He realized how he was accommodating his clients because of his need to be accommodated by me. It was at this time that he was able to move ahead in his sessions and treatment with his clients.

Ms. E. is another supervisee who is in her late thirties. She has been in private practice for about five years. Like Mr. B., she had conflicts about her clients. She, too, felt she gave her clients so much and they didn't appreciate her. When I tried to discuss her need to give and to feel appreciated she couldn't hear me. I explained that our work isn't about giving, and I shared my observations that she spilled over, was too active, and worked too hard, but my words didn't sink in. It wasn't until I focused on my own countertransference feelings that I realized how hard I was working with her, and how much energy and emotion I had invested in keeping her satisfied. I knew my countertransference feelings were the key to how she felt with her clients. Once I was no longer emotionally involved in keeping her happy and wasn't hooked into her, balance and boundaries were reestablished. I could then help her to understand how excessively emotionally involved she was with her clients, how her need to give advice and to rescue them was not only not helpful but actually obstructing the treatment.

My relationships with both Mr. B. and Ms. E. were significant. Understanding my countertransference feelings freed up our work together, which then helped them to move on with their clients.

As I have reflected on Strean's contributions to supervision, particularly his attempts to ensure a more egalitarian atmosphere between supervisor and supervisee, I began to consider where his concepts can be more usefully applied. They are currently being utilized in psychoanalytic training institutes as well as in the supervision of private practitioners. I look forward to the day when the two-person model that Dr. Strean advocates for supervison will be used where it is needed most—in social agencies and mental health centers.

As Strean (1982) himself suggested, supervision in agencies and mental health centers is often too authoritarian and undynamic. Consequently, supervisor and supervisee can often unwittingly take flight from the clients. When the supervisor's countertransference becomes an essential discussing point in the supervision, clients, therapists, and supervisors will be better able to see themselves and each other as more human and more humane.

REFERENCE

Strean, H. (1982). *Controversies in Psychotherapy*. Metuchen, NJ: Scarecrow Press.

6

The Post-Graduation Syndrome: Psychoanalysts Regress as They Cope with Stress

It has repeatedly been demonstrated that no therapist can help his patients grow beyond the point that the therapist himself has reached. If the therapist has been unable to resolve work inhibitions, marital conflicts, parent–child, or other interpersonal problems of his own, he will be unable to help his patients overcome their anxieties and inhibitions in these areas. Similar to the way therapy of the classical neuroses was made possible by Freud's self-analysis, the extension of psychoanalysis and psychotherapy to practically all human conditions has been made possible by the consistent and deepening analyses of practitioners (Fine 1982).

By now, virtually all psychoanalytically oriented therapists have discarded the medical model of the sick patient who is being treated by the healthy doctor. Rather, they tend to concur with Harry Stack Sullivan who averred that we "are all more human than otherwise" (Sullivan 1962). Just as differences between happy, mature individuals and unhappy, psychotic patients are matters of degree, the differences between the emotional health of patients and therapists are also matters of degree. However, when the patient's emotional maturity is greater than the therapist's, which does occur from time to time, it is, of course, very difficult, if not impossible, for the therapist to help the patient grow appreciably. This phenomenon, incidentally, may account for more premature terminations of therapy than has been recognized.

Dynamically oriented therapists also tend to concur with the notion that the growth of patient and therapist proceeds simultaneously. Practitioners continually report that as they confront their own forbidden wishes, diminish the punitiveness of their own superegos, relinquish pathological and maladaptive defenses, and strengthen their own ego functions, their patients concomitantly report similar growth patterns in themselves. Just as self-aware, mature parents raise self-aware, mature children, the same phenomenon seems to occur in therapist–patient relationships. Those therapists who courageously face themselves are usually the ones who can best provide an enabling atmosphere for their patients to do likewise.

Over the years many writers have argued that one of the impediments to helping practitioners mature to their optimum is the nature of psychoanalytic and psychotherapeutic training programs, which tend to foster too much childish dependency in their candidates and provide too much infantile gratification for them (Ekstein and Wallerstein 1958, Strean 1982). Jacob Arlow (1982) has pointed out that much of psychoanalytic education inadvertently tends to further the candidates' desire to overcome their difficulties by identifying themselves with their own analysts. Furthermore, this tends to be reinforced by the idealization of authority figures, which interferes with the candidates' movement in their personal analyses and with their professional growth. The training, therefore, may not work through the candidates' identifications, with a concomitant development of insight; instead, little is resolved and only the identification takes place. Arlow has also commented on the curricula used in most institutes, which encourage imitation of the master rather than independent and critical examination of the data. Siegfried Bernfeld (1962), although writing years before Arlow, viewed the curricula and the dynamics in training institutes quite similarly to Arlow's formulation.

Leo Rangell (1982) has discussed an aspect of psychoanalytic training that has not been fully considered, namely, a possible destructive result to incomplete resolution of the candidate's negative or positive transference to the training analyst, caused by the unanalyzed oedipal conflict. Rangell suggests that when resolution of a persistently strong negative transference is incomplete, the graduate may displace negative feeling to the analyst's theoretical orientation and repudiate the analyst's and/or the institute's theoretical position. In some cases, this may lead to the formation of a deviant group. Rangell also points out that when the positive transference is unresolved, the graduate may displace the idealization of the analyst to theory and blindly accept everything the analyst espouses without any ability to maintain an independent position. This phenomenon, if not properly understood in the training program, can lead to many difficulties and can jeopardize the future development of psychoanalysis. Rangell also discusses such groups as the Kleinian, Kohutian, Bionian, and Faberian, and shows how, in many of these groups, the existence of the oedipal conflict is completely denied; instead it is acted out in the group formation which promulgates the deviant group.

That psychoanalytic and psychotherapeutic training program and institutes have not resolved some serious problems in their organizational structures is quite apparent. That many graduates of training programs have serious neurotic problems and need further help with their internal psychic organizations is also apparent. However, the only way we can improve our training programs and enhance the work of our practitioners is to constantly examine and reexamine our work culture and better comprehend its conflicts and its dynamics.

This paper is an attempt to offer some additional understanding on how our psychoanalytic and psychotherapeutic training programs tend to intensify and exacerbate conflicts in their candidates. More specifically, I would like to report on the responses of more than a dozen graduates of different training institutes who, upon successful completion of their respective programs, all demonstrated rather severe neurotic reactions that interfered with their work with their patients for some time. I would also like to comment on the relationship of these graduates' neurotic responses to some of the dysfunctional aspects of our training programs. All of the graduates I am discussing in this paper were in supervision (or "in control") with me for a minimum of two years and all of them remained in supervision with me for a minimum of one year following the successful completion of their training.

THE POST-GRADUATION SYNDROME: A BRIEF DESCRIPTION

Although the number of the group under examination is small, fourteen to be exact, all of the eight women and six men discussed, upon successful completion of their work from different recognized and well-accepted psychoanalytic institutes, shared very similar reactions. Within two weeks to two months following the successful termination of their training, they all showed in one way or another a lessening of their diagnostic and therapeutic skills, a diminution in their sensitivity to and empathy with patients, a questioning of the efficacy of psychoanalysis as a therapeutic method, a doubting of the benefits of their own personal analysis, and concern with the ability of their supervisor.

Of the fourteen men and women under study, all of them,

after graduation, seriously questioned their own abilities to perform psychoanalytic therapy. Despite the fact that in many contexts and on many occasions they all had demonstrated that they were proficient in understanding and dealing with the complexities and subtleties of transference and resistance phenomena, most of them, after graduation, found it difficult to relate therapeutically to several of their patients and often appeared like beginning therapists when with them. In many cases they offered unnecessary advice to their patients, became overactive in sessions, and in other ways departed from acceptable psychoanalytic procedures. A few became so helpless and so lacking in self-confidence that they began to wonder if they had chosen the right profession.

Although all fourteen men and women had presented a Final Case Presentation to a committee of three or more senior analysts and received unqualified endorsement of their work from them, with no exception, the graduates began to wonder whether the patients they presented to their committees had really made any therapeutic progress. Three of the graduates were absolutely convinced that treatment had not helped their patients at any time, and two were quite certain that their patients had severely regressed and were worse off because of the treatment.

It should be noted that all fourteen graduates had a minimum of fifty supervisory sessions on the case they presented to their committees. Consequently, transference and countertransference issues were discussed in depth in their supervisory conferences; resistances, counterresistances, dreams, technical procedures, and many other aspects of psychoanalytic theory and practice were also examined and discussed in detail. Despite this, after the candidates' successful presentations to their committees, in time they all appeared very lacking in confidence and frequently seemed ignorant about many elementary notions of psychoanalysis.

With the aid of their own personal analyses and supervision the graduates were eventually able to master their professional crises and resolve their conflicts. Because of the focus on this presentation, I would like to examine in more detail why fourteen competent people with many years of psychoanalytic education, personal analyses, and supervision, after their graduation from respectable training institutes, all regressed for several weeks, and occasionally for several months, and appeared like wobbly beginners.

While every therapist, like every human being, develops his own personal and internal drive psychology, his own ego psychology, and his own special object relations and self-psychology (Pine 1985), for purposes of this discussion I am dividing the group of fourteen men and women into several categories. These categories, although somewhat arbitrary, attempt to focus on the major dynamic issue involved in the candidates' professional crises. It should be mentioned, however, that the four categories: (1) oedipal conflicts, (2) separation-individuation conflicts, (3) superego-punishment, and (4) wishes to regress, are not mutually exclusive. It was quite possible that a graduate who showed many oedipal conflicts operating in his neurotic reaction to graduation, could also be suffering from separation-individuation conflicts or wanting superego punishment or wishing to regress. However, each category calls attention to what appeared to be the most salient dynamic issue in provoking the graduates' professional crises.

Category 1—Oedipal Conflicts

A number of the graduates who were reacting very negatively to their patients, to their supervisor, and to psychoanalytic theory and practice, were suffering from unresolved oedipal conflicts. It was as if their graduation unconsciously appeared to them as a puberty rite and they could now use their increased potency and their elevated status to eradicate their parental figures, much like young people do in a primal horde. For them to go on accepting psychoanalytic theory and practice was equivalent to being submissive children who did not have identities of their own. Consequently, they took on what Erikson (1950) has called *negative identities* and opposed much of what their mentors stood for. They questioned traditional psychoanalytic theory and practice and rebelled against psychoanalytic tenets they had been constructively utilizing for years. In several cases they were consciously fighting their analysts and supervisors intensely and in two cases the graduates were convinced that the latter were jealous of them.

Ms. L. Paul, a married woman of forty, had been an excellent student throughout her seven years of training at a psychoanalytic institute.

She had completed a successful personal analysis, responded very positively to all of her supervisors while in training, and was well liked by her peers and teachers. In addition to being well regarded as a professional, Ms. Paul impressed most of her mentors and peers as a happily married mother of two children.

During her year of supervision with me, Ms. Paul demonstrated an excellent grasp of psychoanalytic concepts, was continually empathetic with the male patient she used for her control case, and consistently responded positively to supervisory direction and guidance.

The patient she presented to her committee had, through her help, shown a great deal of positive movement in his work life and in his love life, and her committee lauded her work and her case presentation.

Inasmuch as Ms. Paul found her supervision to be a constructive and enhancing experience professionally, she wanted to remain in it after graduation so that she could discuss more of her cases in depth. After about a month of doing this, Ms. Paul began to tell me that the patient we had been working on during the past year was regressing. He was showing work problems, having sexual difficulties, and was quite depressed. Eventually she went on to point out that maybe he had never made any progress at all and that maybe she should stop treating him altogether. This was in spite of the fact that prior to her presentation her patient was heading toward marriage and moving ahead on his job.

When it became clear to me that Ms. Paul had an investment in viewing my work with her as a failure, as well as viewing her own work with her patient as a failure, I shared this impression of mine with her. Being a responsible, mature, and very insightful person, Ms. Paul was eventually able to bring out that upon graduation she felt smug and superior to her own analyst, who was a woman. Her new status as a full-fledged psychoanalyst reactivated memories of her own mother, toward whom she had felt quite competitive, and at times with whom she felt like an oedipal victor.

Ms. Paul was able to recognize that her success with her case, as well as having me as a supportive father figure, intensified her oedipal conflicts. Her need to believe she had not helped her patient was an overdetermined reaction. By failing with her case, she could knock her "mother-analyst" and say, "psychoanalysis is worthless"; she could also punish herself for having her "father supervisor's" support, which unconsciously was experienced as forbidden incest.

Category 2—Separation-Individuation Conflicts

While graduation conjures up associations of being equal to or surpassing parents and therefore can reactive oedipal conflicts, it is also a time of separating from parental figures. Consequently, fears of autonomy, anxiety about cutting the cord, lost opportunities to lean and learn, and conflicts around dependency can and often do emerge.

All of the graduates under examination experienced some anxiety about being on their own and this was one of the reasons they all elected to stay in supervision beyond graduation, even though there was no formal requirement for them to do so. While all of the graduates felt some discomfort about being autonomous practitioners, several were extremely frightened about the prospect. Said one graduate, "The idea of being completely on my own without supervision and without analysis scares the hell out of me. I can't walk alone." Like some toddlers who cannot tolerate the anxiety of walking alone without being accompanied by a parental figure, many graduates from analytic institutes seem to feel the same way. And, just as many children cannot cope with separation from their parents because it feels as if their parents are dead, graduates, by the same token, can feel the same way about their mentors because of their death wishes toward them.

As graduates talked about their relationships to their training institutes, particularly when they shared information about their relationships with their analysts, teachers, and supervisors, it appeared that many of them were involved in a strong symbiosis with their institutes. Separation from their institutes was equivalent to mutual death—a frightening prospect, and hence, the candidates had a strong wish to maintain ties to their institutes. One way of maintaining the ties was to try to show their supervisor and themselves that they knew very little about psychoanalysis and that they needed much more supervision and much more personal analysis before they could consider being on their own.

Mr. N. Lee was a forty-four-year-old married graduate who had spent approximately nine years in analytic training. Although most of his instructors and supervisors spoke well of him and referred to his strong motivation to learn, his dedication to his patients, and his absorption with the psychoanalytic literature, a few noted that he could also be ingratiating on occasion, often obsessive, and reluctant to accept criticism from supervisors from time to time.

In his control work Mr. Lee, though defensive on occasion, was ready to learn most of the time and did very successful analytic work with a young woman teacher who had many sexual and interpersonal problems with men. After some initial anxiety, which made him somewhat inhibited for a short while, he did write up his Final Case clearly and thoroughly, showing good diagnostic understanding and much sensitivity to transference and countertransference phenomena, resistances, dreams, history, and other salient dimensions of analytic work. Still in analysis, Mr. Lee reported to me that he was able to use some of his analytic sessions to reduce his anxiety about his Final Case Presentation.

Two weeks after Mr. Lee successfully presented his Final Case and was praised highly by the committee members, he became very agitated, depressed, and helpless in his supervisory sessions. He found it difficult to use psychoanalytic concepts in the constructive way to which he had been accustomed, but, instead, stammered and hedged. He became very withdrawn in his work with the patient he had presented for his Final Case and was quite withdrawn with his other patients as well.

When I noted with Mr. Lee how upset he had become since graduation, his first response was, "I don't feel like a graduate. I don't feel like an analyst. Maybe it's a dream." Further discussion with Mr. Lee revealed that he felt very frightened of growing up. "I look at you as a benign big brother who takes good care of me. The idea of finishing up at the Institute threatens that. I worried my head off that maybe you would tell me I should try it on my own." He went on to share with me some childhood experiences in which he not only felt abandoned by his mother and an aunt but, helpless, *was* abandoned by them. Just as he felt resourceless, helpless, and hopeless at the age of 6 when his mother and aunt were not available for him, Mr. Lee experienced the termination of his analytic training as an acute loss and as a potential abandonment. It took him some time in his own personal analysis to diminish the trauma that graduation had held for him.

Category 3—Superego Punishment

Anyone who has practiced psychoanalytic therapy cannot fail to note in his daily work constant expressions of superego punishment. Some examples are: "I don't have a right to pleasure"; "I feel guilty when I achieve something"; "I feel when I get something for myself, I'm depriving someone else." Frequently patients project their superegos onto their therapists and say, "You will criticize me for this"; "You will punish me for that"; "I get the feeling, although you haven't said anything about it, that you don't like me."

Very often people seek therapy primarily because they are dimly aware of how punitive they are with themselves. Indeed, one of the major differences between individuals who are drawn to therapy and those who shun it is that the former are quite guilt-ridden and more willing to acknowledge their guilt rather than rationalize it or deny it (Fine 1982). Usually the person who fights therapy, whether he is a patient or not, ascribes the causes of his unhappiness to others and finds it difficult to assume responsibility for his own plights.

Inasmuch as people who become therapists usually fantasize that their choice of profession will help them resolve their own neuroses, that is, their choice of work can be a disguised way of receiving therapy, we would expect therapists to have many guilts of their own. And when they accomplish something as noteworthy as graduating from an analytic institute, we would expect them to feel quite guilty—and indeed, they do. Virtually every one of the fourteen individuals in this study voiced some guilt about being made a full-fledged psychoanalyst. Statements on this theme were many: "I don't believe I should be in the same league as you and my analyst"; "I feel like an impostor"; "I feel I got away with something"; "In some ways I feel like a crook, calling myself an analyst"; "Sometimes I think I'm living in a dream and I'm going to wake up and find out I'm still a student."

As analysts know, when an individual feels that he deserves punishment, he feels guilty about thoughts, fantasies, feelings, or deeds. Termination of analytic training for most of the graduates induced guilt because they seemed to experience graduation as "a hostile triumph," "a sexual seduction," "an oedipal victory," or in a few cases like "a crime" for which they had to be punished.

> Dr. B. Miles was a forty-two-year-old married man with two children, who had been a student in a training insti-ute for over ten years. A very likable man who induced many affectionate feelings in those around him, at times he seemed mildly depressed and somewhat unassertive. Nonetheless, he successfully completed a personal analy-sis, did satisfactory work in his courses, and wrote a very clear Final Case Presentation that demonstrated good understanding of psychoanalytic theory and treatment.
>
> The case Dr. Miles had in control was a married man involved in a severe sadomasochistic struggle with his wife. Dr. Miles was able to help his patient lessen the severity of his marital conflicts, and during treatment the patient was also able to enhance himself professionally in a major way. The patient's sense of impotence and helplessness diminished and his self-esteem and self-image grew.
>
> Dr. Miles was unanimously passed by his committee

and warmly endorsed to be a member of the analytic society affiliated with the institute he attended. While he felt pleased and was exuberant about his achievements, within three weeks after graduation he appeared morose, confused, and very uncertain of himself in his supervisory conferences. The patient he had used for his presentation, as far as Dr. Miles was concerned, had not made much progress at all. Dr. Miles felt he had not really dealt with the patient's resistances, the transference was hardly considered, and the patient's marriage was still very chaotic.

When it was pointed out to Dr. Miles that he seemed to be feeling very upset about himself and his work ever since he successfully completed his training and was passed by his committee, he became quite thoughtful. As he thought about what was going on with him, he shared with me the reflection that he had spent a lot of time in his own personal analysis working on his self-hatred. He mentioned a rather persistent dream during his analysis in which he found himself successfully dribbling a basketball all the way down the full basketball court, only to miss an easy lay-up shot at the end. Clearly, Dr. Miles was acting out this dream in his response to graduation but not letting himself feel that he had achieved anything substantial, even though he had successfully "carried the ball" and competently finished his training.

Further discussion with Dr. Miles revealed that his own father had not achieved very much. Consequently, Dr. Miles was unconsciously placing himself in his father's shoes and suffering, instead of enjoying his earned success. Later, when I suggested to Dr. Miles that maybe he was making me his inadequate father who really had not taught him anything very much, he was able to get in touch with his latent hostile transference to me and tie it up with material he had worked on in the past in his own analysis. This enabled him to restore his confidence about his work and helped him to lift his morose demeanor.

Category 4—Wishes to Regress

Just as every analyst constantly witnesses patients seeking punishment, he also notes in virtually every one of them a wish to regress. Regression is so frequently seen in practice because all patients at times find their present circumstances anxiety provoking. Therefore, it is easier for them to return to older forms of gratification that pose less danger. Just as children who find toilet-training very upsetting and conflictful may return to older patterns of behavior and wet their beds and suck their thumbs, adults do something similar when the going gets tough. For example, when adult patients cannot cope with competitive fantasies toward their therapists, they often regress and talk about homosexual desires and dependency yearnings instead. And when more mature sexual desires are frightening to them, they can regress to the position of a clinging child.

As graduation symbolizes adulthood for most individuals, it should not surprise us that every one of the fourteen therapists under study verbalized wishes to remain a student and not graduate. At least eight of the fourteen said the following to me: "I know that you're not used to having your students flunk their Final Case Presentation but I'll be the first!" After graduation most of them talked about how much gratification they derived from being a student and how uncomfortable they were about giving up the student role. Said one typical graduate, "As a student you're taken care of. As a graduate you're out in the cold!" Another graduate stated, "It feels like being dumped in the water and being told to swim before you feel ready."

Inasmuch as the autonomous, independent status of a full-fledged analyst was so frightening to all of the graduates, virtually all digressed and regressed from the rigorous discipline of doing psychoanalytic therapy. A few took long vacations at a time they normally would be working. Several began to flirt with doing other kinds of treatment—family therapy, marriage counseling, and so on—and all of them became quite needy in supervision. They asked for explanations to questions that in the past they really knew how to answer themselves. They couldn't figure out the dynamics of several patients whose dynamics they had figured out some time ago, and they were perplexed about how to resolve patients' resistances that in the past were not difficult for them to resolve. Suddenly they found many of their patients in crisis and they needed their supervisor to bail them out. Several made phone calls to me in between their supervisory sessions for assistance with cases, something they rarely had to do in the past.

> Ms. A. Smith, a married woman in her late forties, had been an excellent student during her eight years of psychoanalytic training. All of her teachers commented on her warm disposition, her dedication to her patients, her intelligence, and her marked ability to learn quickly. She also impressed mentors and peers as happily married and enjoying her two children.
>
> Ms. Smith had no difficulty writing her Final Case Presentation or presenting it to her committee. The patient she had in control was a single woman in her early thirties who had a lot of sexual and other interpersonal difficulties with men. Ms. Smith did very effective analytic work with her patient and dealt very well with the latter's positive and negative transference reactions and with her different forms of resistance. Her committee was very impressed with her excellent presentation, which demonstrated solid analytic work.
>
> Although Ms. Smith had impressed her teachers, supervisors, and peers as a competent practitioner, within

two weeks after her successful presentation, she regressed to a level that made her appear like a beginner. She "forgot" all the theory she had learned, could not understand what her patients were talking about, and felt that she had no treatment skills. In addition, she appeared mildly depressed, quite helpless, and very much lacking in self-confidence. For several weeks she called me in between supervisory sessions for assistance.

The dramatic shift in Ms. Smith's mood was so clearly related to completing her training that she had no difficulty seeing for herself that graduation was very threatening to her. Graduation stimulated internal demands to be omnipotent. She experienced her male analyst and me as omnipotent phalluses and felt that she was now required to assume this lofty status. The wish, while strong, appeared so ominous and terrifying to her that she regressed to being a helpless little girl who needed a strong parental figure to take care of her.

Ms. Smith's regressed behavior, which lasted for a few months, was intense and pervasive. She was still in analysis and was able to work on and eventually lessen the need for it.

DISCUSSION

While we have been dealing with a small sample of analysts-in-training who worked with only one supervisor, there appear, nonetheless, to be several implications and hypotheses that evolve from this study. One of the most obvious findings is that psychoanalysts have difficulty relinquishing their student role. All of the men and women in this study functioned extremely well as therapists as long as they were students. Becoming "psychoanalytic adults" seemed to frighten them, and all of them in one way or another wanted to continue to lean on parental figures.

The attraction to the student role and the dependency gratification that it offers may suggest something about psychoanalysts, at least about the psychoanalysts in this study. Perhaps those attracted to the profession of psychoanalysis, a profession that requires one person to be dependent on another, offers analysts vicarious gratifications. As they nurture and take care of others, they are taking care of themselves. However, to just take care of others is insufficient for many analysts. They seem to want for themselves what they give to their patients and if they feel there is a possibility that they will not get it, they resent their patients and move away from them emotionally. It will be recalled that when the analysts we have been discussing were undergoing stress and were worried about cutting the cord from their own parental figures, their patients were concomitantly complaining about their treatment. This suggests that for many analysts, perhaps for most, if they are not being given to, either in supervision, personal analysis, or somewhere else, such as in marriage or friendship, they cannot consistently give to others therapeutically.

Another application of this study is that analysts seem to have some difficulty enjoying success. The majority of the men and women in this study had trouble accepting an equal status with their supervisors and analysts. Many of them experienced graduation as an oedipal triumph for which they should be punished; consequently, to avoid castration, rejection, or abandonment, they clung to the student role and became childlike. This finding seems to confirm Rangell's (1982) notion that many graduates of psychoanalytic institutes have unresolved oedipal conflicts. It is not known whether those men and women who become psychoanalysts are "more oedipal" than those who choose other fields, but we may hypothesize, nonetheless, that some of their unresolved oedipal conflicts may have something to do with the nature of analytic training. Most analytic students are in analysis with faculty members of the institute they attend. Often they see their analysts in the classroom, at meetings, and elsewhere. Is it more difficult for an analyst-in-training to face his murderous and competitive fantasies toward one who is on the faculty of the institute he highly cathects? In some analytic institutes, the analyst decides when and if the candidate can take courses in the institute. Does this not influence the candidate and induce him to hold back oedipal fantasies and perhaps other material as well? While analysts-in-training, like all patients, make their analysts and supervisors superego figures, do not the latter realistically slip into a superego role?

The nature of our training system in most psychoanalytic institutes might induce many analysts-in-training to comply with their mentors' psychoanalytic orientation and squelch their hostility toward their supervisors and analysts when they disagree with them. Perhaps a great deal of repressed hostility comes out at graduation when it may be a little safer for it to be discharged. Yet, even at graduation, as our vignettes show, the rage, competition, and murder are expressed in a disguised form. It was still too threatening, even after graduation, for many of the men and women to bring out their negative feelings toward their mentors directly.

While writing this paper, I became aware of how in my role as a supervisor I "helped" my students to hold back their resentment while they were in "control" and consequently "helped" them regress after graduation. During the preparation of students for Final Case Presentation, I customarily try to predict questions that are going to be asked of them. Having been affiliated with psychoanalytic institutes for close to thirty years and knowing how my psychoanalytic colleagues think, I find that most of my predictions do come true. As a result, students are prepared for the questions and also have the answers at their fingertips. While this can help them pass their Final Case Presentation with a fair amount of ease, it can also make them feel that they are merely mimicking me, incorporating me, and mirroring me but not using their own ego strengths sufficiently. Having passed the test, they may think they have been pushed through the institute rather than having independently passed, and hence, they may resent me. Not able to deal with resenting somebody who has helped them so much, they push the hatred underground, only to have it come out later in disguised, self-destructive, and masochistic forms of behavior. My own stance just referred to might be considered an example of what Arlow (1982), Bernfeld (1962), Ekstein and Wallerstein (1958) and others (Strean 1982) have referred to as the infantilization of analytic students, where too much dependency gratification is provided, with insufficient amount of autonomy fostered. There are probably other examples of this overencouragement of dependency that can be found in my own supervisory and analytic work and in that of other psychoanalysts.

In examining the reactions of our graduates, particularly how they all reacted negatively to their analysts, supervisors, and the psychoanalytic profession in general, I am reminded of something similar to Freud's notion of the "negative therapeutic reaction" (1923). Here, Freud talked about the many patients who could verbalize all the explanations and interpretations, but went on to feel unhappy and uncomfortable in their lives. Freud felt that what kept these patients from moving forward was their punitive superegos—the internalized voices of their parents.

In looking at the candidates' negative reactions more closely, analysts have found that those individuals who exhibit this type of behavior are harboring unconscious resentment and revenge toward their therapists. Reuben Fine (1982), in discussing these individuals, points out that many of them are from homes in which the parents could relate to them only when they were young and dependent. Once the children reached adolescence, the threat of the children's emancipation was so overpowering to the parents that they curbed their children's growth and compounded their children's revenge. How much parental figures in psychoanalytic institutes are unconsciously interfering with their students' and/or analysands' emancipation is a question that deserves much more serious study than has been given to it. Are analytic students rewarded for compliance more than we realize? How comfortable are analytic teachers and supervisors when they are opposed?

Just as patients cannot be helped beyond where their analysts have reached, psychoanalytic mentors must examine and reexamine how much they are trying to maintain themselves as controlling, omnipotent parents who wish to make their students and patients miniatures of themselves. They have to examine and reexamine how much dependency and imitation they foster in their analytic curricula and what they can do to promote more creative, independent thinking. Maybe more students should be rewarded and praised for questioning their mentors than they usually are. Maybe more attention has to be given to the extra-analytic contacts that transpire between analyst and student and what impact this has on the student's growth. Maybe senior analysts have to convene more often among themselves to examine their countertransference problems with students who are in supervision and in analysis with them.

The questions, findings, and implications of this paper will not be resolved quickly. However, they demand attention, and soon!

REFERENCES

Arlow, J. (1982). Psychoanalytic education: a psychoanalytic perspective. *Annual of Psychoanalysis* 10:5–20.
Bernfeld, S. (1962). On psychoanalytic education. *Psychoanalytic Quarterly* 31:453–482.
Ekstein, R., and Wallerstein, R. S. (1958). *The Teaching and Learning of Psychotherapy*. New York: Basic Books.
Erikson, E. (1950). *Childhood and Society*. New York: Norton.

Fine, R. (1981). *The Psychoanalytic Vision.* New York: Free Press.

―――― (1982). *The Healing of the Mind,* 2nd ed. New York: Free Press.

Freud, S. (1920). Beyond the pleasure principle. *Standard Edition* 18:1–65.

―――― (1923). The ego and the id. *Standard Edition* 19:12–68.

Pine, F. (1985). *Development Theory and Clinical Process.* New Haven, CT: Yale University Press.

Rangell, L. (1982). Transference to theory: the relationship of psychoanalytic education to the analyst's relationship to psychoanalysis. *Annual of Psychoanalysis* 10:29–56.

Strean, H. (1982). *Controversy in Psychotherapy.* Metuchen, NJ: Scarecrow Press.

Sullivan, H. S. (1962). *Schizophrenia as a Human Process.* New York: Norton.

Discussion:
Post-Graduation Syndrome:
The Shadow of the Object

James W. Hull

What we cannot reach by flying, we can reach by limping.
It is no sin to limp.

(Freud, 1920)

Dr. Strean's paper is an interesting and careful consideration of a topic that receives little attention within the psychoanalytic community, probably because it makes everyone so uncomfortable. In discussing what happens to graduates after they complete their training, and what problems they have due to conflicts not resolved during their training analyses, Strean is peering behind the façade of psychoanalytic training and asking some tough questions. How well analyzed is the successful graduate? What about the conflicts that have been left unresolved? How will they affect the new graduate and his work with future patients? How do graduates go about completing the work of their own analyses? Do training programs themselves contribute to unresolved conflicts by fostering dependency and rewarding identification and imitation rather than independent critical thinking? Does this interfere with the growth of psychoanalysis as a field, as Rangell (1982) has suggested?

Probably all analysts begin their training with the hope of being fully analyzed. With their core issues resolved, they hope to be able to offer their patients the highest level of care. Despite regular emphasis by training staff on the "interminable" nature of analysis, and reminders about the need to occasionally go back for further analysis and/or supervision, institutes also covertly support the view that their graduates will be fully analyzed, priding themselves on the thoroughness of their training and the quality of the practitioners they turn out. This is part of the culture of psychoanalysis, the ego ideal that we all share. It also reflects prominent values in our larger culture, especially the pursuit of perfection. We barrage our youth with the need to achieve, make money, and be perfect, in the process causing them to lose a sense of their own vulnerabilities and essential humanness. In these booming economic times, people demand quick, discrete, warrantied results, and are prepared to search for blame and sue when things don't live up to expectations. Psychiatry has embraced this view in its search for the perfect prescription drug. In our consumer-oriented society a company would go out of business if it acknowledged and openly talked about turning out a good but a partially complete product, a product that still needed work and might never perform to its full potential. It is no wonder that psychoanalytic training programs don't often talk about how complete their training really is, how they may actually inhibit the growth of their candidates, or how their graduates' unresolved conflicts affect future patients.

Of course, patients do not get better or grow emotionally from prescription drugs, and analysts are not like automobiles, issued with a warranty and the possibility of a recall should future defects be uncovered. Ours is a much more humble and human enterprise, messy; unpredictable; fraught with uncertainties, failures, and limited results; but also sometimes yielding spectacular, breathtaking successes when people are helped to change their lives in ways they never thought possible. Strean embraces this human endeavor, asking the difficult questions, and courageously encouraging us to keep trying to understand the experience of our patients and ourselves.

But what about Herb's own work? Do his analysands go through post-graduation syndrome?

Because I had the good fortune of completing a ten-year analysis with him, I am in a position to provide a powerful illustration of the phenomena he describes. My analysis with Herb began shortly after my father's early death from heart disease. During much of the analysis I struggled to come to terms with my father's emotional unavailability, as well as his intermittent rages that felt so dangerous. I came to understand my first choice of career, mathematics, as an attempt to navigate the separation of adolescence through the creation of an ordered and predictable world that was free of my father's and my own rage. Only much later, in graduate school, did I move back toward people in a search for more meaning in my life. Throughout my analytic journey Herb was consistently there for me and provided me the help and nurturance I had not received from my father.

But of course it was hard for me to fight with him. How could I express rage at a person who had given me so much, who was one of the smartest people I knew, and who in many ways had been a better father than my own? I struggled with this issue and made progress, increasingly voicing my resentments, but I probably never was truly comfortable with my hatred and death wishes toward Herb. In my mind this felt too much like my own father's rages and was linked to death—my father's, Herb's, or my own. The first sign of future trouble was the way I ended my analysis. Herb and I both agreed that I was ready to stop, but I insisted on terminating immediately rather than following his recommendation to continue for another few months until the summer break. Why, after ten years, could I not wait a few more months? The answer lies in Herb's paper.

In looking back I believe that my relationship with Herb, especially in the early stages of the analysis, followed the pattern of primitive identification described by Schafer (1994) in his analysis of the work of contemporary Kleinians. Herb was a source of such nurturance, he was the father that I had longed for, and I sought to incorporate him completely. I felt he had all the answers about how to practice psychoanalysis and I wanted to be just like him. I consciously tried to conduct myself in sessions the way I imagined he would. I adopted his policies about payment and missed sessions. Even the message on my answering machine sounded like his. As Freud wrote, "The shadow of the object falls across the ego . . ."

Although imitation and identification can be a valuable early stage of learning, problems arise when issues about anger and aggression haven't been worked through. As Freud described, when the object is lost, through death (or in this case the ending of an analysis), the introject becomes the target of the unresolved aggression. In effect the person goes to war against himself. After completing my analysis I began to feel burdened by the need to work exactly like Herb. I remember one day when I had the flu and wanted to cancel my sessions, but then realized with shock that in ten years Herb had never once canceled a session because of routine illness. This was terribly frustrating because I knew I never could live up to such a standard, and I wasn't sure that I wanted to.

This unresolved hatred toward Herb (and ultimately my father) affected my feelings about being an analyst and the details of my work with patients. I began to doubt that I could be successful, I wondered whether I had what it took, and I suspected that psychoanalysis might be a sham profession. I had a great deal of difficulty keeping track of money my patients owed me, which is quite an accomplishment for a former mathematician. As I struggled to cope with this anger triggered by my separation from Herb, I again tried the solution that had worked in adolescence. I changed jobs, making a career move away from clinical work toward statistics (mathematics again!) that lasted for five years. The graduates in Herb's case studies should not feel too bad if they felt lost "for several weeks, and occasionally for several months" due to their regressions at the end of training. My detour was a much grander voyage!

An interesting thing happened during this career detour, however. I continued to treat patients, thinking of it as a sideline that gave me pleasure instead of my primary job. I began canceling sessions when I was ill, and in general did things my own way. At first I was more comfortable treating a different type of patient than I imagined Herb worked with. I became more spontaneous during sessions, and when a patient suddenly left me I didn't worry too much about it, feeling it was as much her loss as mine. Interestingly enough, the work went well and my practice slowly grew. I began to comfortably think of myself as an analyst again. As the shadow of the object faded I reclaimed my sense of myself as a separate person and analyst, connected to Herb but not fused with him.

The resolution of these issues also was moved forward by Herb's struggle with heart disease and his openness in talking to me about it. I remember going to see him after his heart attack and having him laugh when I said I just needed to check in and see that he was okay. Unconsciously I think I was checking to see whether my aggressive fantasies had destroyed him, and was reassured that he wasn't threatened by them and was able to talk about his experience nondefensively. His openness and his willingness to share his countertransference feelings helped me understand and accept my own unconscious fantasies toward him. If he had responded like Freud's surgeon I would have been in serious trouble and would have had much more difficulty finding my way out of the woods. Another analyst, who defensively assumed a neutral stance, might have helped me stay lost.

It is no sin to limp.

REFERENCES

Freud, S. (1920). Beyond the pleasure principle. *Standard Edition* 18:1–119.

Rangell, L. (1982). Transference to theory: the relationship of psychoanalytic education to the analyst's relationship to psychoanalysis. *The Annual of Psychoanalysis* 10:29–56.

Schafer, R. (1994). The contemporary Kleinians of London. *Psychoanalytic Quarterly* 63:409–432.

Discussion:
The Regressive Pull

Angelo Smaldino

A ll that is involved in psychoanalytic training, from personal analysis to supervision, to control analysis, to final case presentation, to graduation, is characterized by an inevitable and necessary process of maturation and growth. This journey, colored by a desire for, and expectations of progress, also contains a pull towards regression. It is the back and forth of any emotional journey, where the presence of new discoveries challenges old adaptations and paves the way for new ones. As old adaptations begin to wobble, anxiety and excitement emerge at the threshold of new possibilities.

It goes without saying that the entire process, which characterizes the movement toward new and more effective ways to adapt to life's challenges, is burdened or facilitated by the quality of previous experiences. More specifically, the individual movement toward separation-individuation, with the internalized quality of self and object representation and object relationships, represents the blueprint that will greatly affect the never-ending process of growth.

It is in this context that Dr. Strean frames the regressive pull observed in recently graduated psychoanalysts. In discussing the graduate's crisis he talks of the wish to regress and he discusses superego conflicts, superego punishment, and separation-individuation conflicts. His paper is cogent, rich with insights and generous in the thought-provoking quality of his presentation.

I would like to present some additional thoughts related to the process of individuation. There is an aspect of the latter part of training that is conflictual for some candidates, the adaptation to which profoundly affects the process that leads to graduation and to the subsequent crisis that Strean describes in his paper. The latter phase of psychoanalytic training is characterized by two control analyses. It is expected that supervision will concentrate on the candidate's work with the control patient who is to be seen at least three times per week on the couch. The candidate is often required to present verbatim sessions to his supervisor. Even when there is more flexibility, the expectation is for a very detailed account of what transpired during the analytic session, not only in terms of the patient's production, but also in terms of the candidate's input, including motivations and reasons for that input. This required aspect of training can set up a potential sense of rigidity for some candidates with consequent rupture in the quality of the learning process.

The issue at hand here is the pattern of learning, the pattern of teaching, and the consequent quality of fit between the two. I do not know how often teachers and supervisors ask themselves whether the type of interactions they have with the candidate may actually foster subterfuges, may stress expression of false self, may further consolidate maladaptive patterns of coping, and may limit expression of creativity. One may object that these are issues that should be brought up and resolved in one's own personal analysis. While I agree that that is the place for exploration, understanding, and resolution of the above, I also believe that the supervisor or the teacher who ignores those issues is colluding with the candidate's old and conflicted individuation problems. It can at times be an even more complicated process because the teacher or supervisor may, through the candidate, express old and not fully resolved conflicts of his own toward the institute in particular and authority in general. Furthermore, it is not unusual that the candidate may find himself to be part of a collusion between divergent narcissistic needs of the analyst and the supervisor. He may become the vehicle through which the supervisor may express his own competitive and/or grandiose feelings. It may happen that the supervisor actively, though subtly, fosters the candidate's resentment toward specific guidelines of the institute, or toward specific attitudes of the candidate's own analyst. It may also happen that the supervisor may passively watch the candidate's entanglement in those positions without facilitating a curiosity that the candidate may utilize for further exploration in his own personal analytic work.

Though it is true that the teaching–learning interaction often evolves in very productive ways that facilitate the resolution of conflicts and thus fosters further growth, what I am exploring here are those aspects of interaction that may contribute to the later regression illustrated by Strean. It is a reality, although, it is hoped, not a very recurrent one, that some candidates will report to their supervisor not only what happened in the sessions with their control patient, but also what they thought should have happened. In these cases the reporting is mostly aimed at pleasing the supervisor by becoming an expression of what the candidate has already learned about the supervisor's orientation and expectations, rather than the candidate's own evolving convictions and doubts. Another potential difficulty is the candidate's concern that the analytic patient may reduce the number of sessions or leave treatment, thus jeopardizing the candidate's ability to complete the requirements for graduation. This anxiety may contribute to the candidate's tendency not to do anything that he thinks might antagonize his patient or cause him to leave treatment. If the candidate is unable to discuss his concerns with the supervisor, and if the supervisor does not pick up on those concerns, the entire teaching process will be askew, and the candidate may be left feeling that to implement some of what the supervisor is communicating may mean losing the patient.

Certainly these difficulties are often recognized and discussed in supervision. Thus they become opportunities for reevaluating the teaching–learning patterns, and for encouraging attention to conflictual issues to be addressed in analysis. Yet, besides the candidate's own characterological issues, the reality of the institute's politics may also contribute to a tacit collusion between teacher and student, supervisee and supervisor. In fact it is not unusual to find (1) divergent theoretical orientations among institute members, sometimes with insidious conflicts between them, (2) power struggles for different positions within the institute, (3) spelled-out but not necessarily agreed-upon requirements for supervision, teaching, and graduation, and (4) teaching methods and attitudes that contribute to the candidate's doubts about purposes and goals, and that may at times encourage subterfuge and lies. For instance, the final case can be presented with the committee under the assumption that the patient was seen in accordance with the requirements spelled out by the institute regarding frequency and use of the couch. Whatever the difference between what is required and what is presented, it certainly reflects the candidate's complex transference to the institute and those who have been intimately involved in his training. Further, it points to patterns of adaptation that may have been problematic and that will continue to exercise their influence after graduation. In those families where parental rigidity seems to be sovereign, children may develop strategies to get their way even as they seem to be compliant. Furthermore, if the rigidity is coupled with the inability to communicate, and with an expectation of silent acceptance of the rules, then it is likely that individuation will take place in an aggressive, defiant way. It is as if only through defiance or dramatic rupture can one hope to gain individuation.

After graduation the candidate has the opportunity to transcend those limitations that may have interfered with his ability to express his own individual orientation and style. Thus regression in new psychoanalysts may represent a necessary step in the development of their individuality as analysts. What I wished to stress here is the collusion that may take place during psychoanalytic training between the institute and its representatives on the one hand, and the candidate with his own patterns of adaptation on the other. The quality of this relationship, while colored by previous patterns of adaptation, also profoundly affects the ongoing process of individuation. Hurn (1970), in discussing the termination phase of analysis, called attention to adolescent conflicts over independence, which may be overlooked during the termination phase. I suggest that the termination phase of analytic training contains issues related to adolescent developmental struggles for independence that become recapitulated, and that may add to the difficult though exciting transition from candidate to graduate. I further suggest that not enough attention is paid to the demands for conformity to requirements and to the ways that some candidates deal with them within the learning atmosphere of the institute.

The conscious and unconscious resentment that ensues, the anxiety about one's ability as an analyst, the anxiety about meeting the requirements that will finally end a long training that has required a great deal of emotional and financial energies, all may contribute to a regressive pull, and to a reactivation of the adolescent wish for independence with the related old conflicts and old attempts at resolution. Unless analytic candidates and their mentors deal with the conflicts enumerated by Strean, regression will be inevitable after graduation. Anna Freud (1936) said that the ego cannot be studied when it is in harmony with the id, the superego, and the outside world; it reveals its nature when there is disharmony among the psychic institutions. During training, the effort for apparent harmony takes up some of the candidate's psychic energy, while in reality the ego is in disarray. After graduation, the disharmony now appears more clearly. The candidate feels his own isolation, and he experiences the freedom to feel the tension associated with his previous need to adapt to situations that required a compromise he had not been fully aware of, or not felt fully free to make. This now-felt disharmony might take the form of a temporary regression. Yet this phase for these new analysts may be the necessary step toward greater ego maturation that may lead to a clearer sense of their own identity as analysts.

REFERENCES

Freud, A. (1936). *The Ego and the Mechanisms of Defence*. New York: International Universities Press, 1966.
Hurn, H. T. (1970). Adolescent transference. *Journal of the American Psychoanalytic Association* 18:342–357.

7

The Patient
Who Would Not
Tell His Name

A cardinal rule of psychoanalytic treatment is that the patient should say everything that comes to mind. Yet, the analysand's conscious withholding of material is a resistance that has confronted every practicing analyst on numerous occasions. While most patients recognize that in order to be helped they must freely offer their thoughts, feelings, fantasies, and dreams, many of them conceal their associations because they fear how the analyst might react or what he might do. This fear frequently involves a projection of the patient's critical superego onto the analyst, who is unconsciously perceived as a disapproving figure (Fine 1982, Freud 1912). However, the motives for keeping secrets from the analyst are valid and often overdetermined.

   The case I will present in this paper is that of a 36-year-old man who was in analysis with me four times a week for close to four years but who had to wait for over a year and a half before he could tell me his name. The analysis of his secret revealed that the reasons for withholding his name from me were overdetermined. Furthermore, after he revealed his name, it became apparent that other conscious secrets were being withheld. As we analyzed the patient's transference responses and resistances, and as I investigated my own countertransference reactions, the analytic work provided suggestions as to why patients consciously hold back material from the analyst.

Mr. A. sought analytic treatment for many reasons. He had just been fired from his job as a clerk and was so depressed that he could not summon up sufficient motivation to seek another job. In addition, he had been suffering from many symptoms for several years. He was plagued by constant insomnia, had peptic ulcers and other gastrointestinal complaints, and suffered from many phobias, such as fear of subways, bridges, small rooms, and cars. He was frequently impotent with his wife and felt there had always been a big distance between them during their marriage. Mr. A. also reported that he could not feel comfortable with his son, aged 5, and his daughter, aged 2, and had little to do with them. Although he had almost always been a good student, he constantly found himself in low-paying jobs and derived little satisfaction from them. "Most of my life," said Mr. A. in his first interview, "I've been a depressed loner."

Mr. A. was the older of two children; he had a sister four years younger. He described his father as a hardworking owner of a candy store. He stated that although his father had little to do with him, he felt pressured and criticized by him on frequent occasions. The father had died when the patient was 14 years old. Mr. A.'s mother was described as alternately seductive and punitive. He envied his sister who got all the attention. At the end of Mr. A.'s first interview, during which he appeared deferential, compliant, and very depressed, he pointed out that he would not be able to be in treatment with me "if you *insist* that I give you my name." When I asked him why he was concerned about my knowing his name, he responded with some irritation, saying, "The government frequently makes check-ups on people, and if they found out that I was in psychoanalytic treatment, I'd never get a job." Again he asked, "Are you gong to *insist* on knowing my name?" I pointed out to Mr. A. that he had used the word "insist" at least twice, and he said, "I'm told psychoanalysts are very insistent people, and I'm wary of them." I suggested that he might wish to have another consultation interview with me so that we could further discuss his doubts about me and about psychoanalytic treatment.

In Mr. A.'s second interview he started the session by telling me that he was pleased that "you didn't insist on getting my name, so I'll try you for a while." When I remained silent, he went on to tell me that he was now worried that I would "insist" that he use the couch. After a brief silence, Mr. A. pointed out that he was feeling an acute back pain that was causing him enormous distress and that he had to sit in an upright position or he would pass out. His associations enabled me to offer the interpretation that he was very worried that I would dominate and control him by insisting that he give me his name and by insisting also that he lie on the couch. The interpretation partially relieved Mr. A. from his back pain, and he ended the second session by saying, "I think we can work something out together. You are not that insistent." But the patient said he had to warn me that while my fee was acceptable, he would prefer paying me in cash rather than a check so that I would not see his name and signature on the checks.

Mr. A. sat up for twenty sessions before using the couch. During this time he spoke of his insecurity on jobs and pointed out that he frequently viewed employers the way he had been experiencing me—as people who *insisted* on dominating and controlling him. He seemed to derive some benefit from an interpretation that the bosses appeared to be reminiscent of his pressuring father, and he was soon able to begin job interviews. Eventually he got a position as an office manager.

After Mr. A. had been on the job for about two weeks, he reported that once again he found himself in arguments and power struggles with supervisors. Although he could now recognize that these interpersonal problems emerged from within him rather than being imposed on him, inasmuch as the identical phenomena had occurred with his father and with me, he felt helpless to do anything about them. I suggested to Mr. A. at this point that he might want to consider using the couch in order to understand better what was unconsciously contributing to his problems with bosses and to his other conflicts.

Although Mr. A. went to the couch and lay down quite compliantly, within two or three sessions he became very suspicious of me and of my motives. He told me that I preferred him to be on the couch so that I could be in a one-upmanship position. He was so glad he had not given me his name because he was now convinced that I would give it to the government agents and get paid for doing so. His paranoid fantasies consumed the analysis for about two months, during which he vehemently described me as an opportunist, a manipulator, a sadist, and probably a homosexual. In his sixth month of treatment, Mr. A. had a dream in which I was yelling at him for his not paying me enough money and for his not being more productive in the analysis. In the dream I was again "insisting" that he tell me more fantasies, more dreams, and more associations. Shortly after the session in which Mr. A. discussed this dream, I told him he felt that I wanted him to be my slave, much as he felt he had to be with his father. The patient agreed with the interpretation and then told me he was convinced that I was involved in psychotherapeutic work so that I could be a slave-master and could sadistically torment my patients.

As Mr. A. "investigated" my motives in becoming a tormenting slave-master, he told me that I was basically a homosexual who was trying to fool the world by acting like a heterosexual. Stated Mr. A. in his eighth month of therapy, "You are essentially a passive man who wants to be fucked up the ass, but are scared to admit it." When I asked Mr. A. what he thought might frighten me about acknowledging my homosexuality, he said, "You like to tease and fool the world. Maybe if you tease somebody long enough, they will rape you in anger—that's what you really want."

Concomitant with Mr. A.'s using his analytic sessions to investigate my homosexuality, he told me how much better his own life was becoming. He was sexually potent with his wife, he was not engaged in struggles with his bosses, and his relationship with his children was much better. The only thing that bothered him about this was that he was convinced that I must be suffering with envy inasmuch as I was a celibate with a homosexual problem while he was enjoying so much sexual pleasure with his wife. Furthermore, Mr. A. felt that as he was achieving pleasure from his work, I also felt envious because I did not seem too happy in my work.

Mr. A. could empathize with my plight because just as I was very jealous of his enjoyable sexual relationship with his wife, he could remember feeling the same way about his parents' sexual relationship. And just as I envied Mr. A.'s success in his job, he could remember when he was a boy and envied his father's popularity and business acumen. For several sessions Mr. A. mocked me, denigrated me, and was contemptuous of me. In one of his dreams during this period he made me a pig with glasses on, trying in vain to do work, but emerging as a failure. In another dream he made me a catcher on a homosexual baseball team. To my query about why a catcher, he answered that he knew I wanted "to sniff the batters' asses and touch their genitals when nobody was looking."

As Mr. A. projected his homosexual wishes onto me and saw that I did not react argumentatively or defensively, he slowly began to identify with my analytic attitude and started to look at his own homosexual fantasies. While tentative and frightened at first, he began to talk of his interest in boys' penises when he was a high school student and showered after gym. When I asked Mr. A. to try to recall his fantasies when he was in the shower with other boys, he spoke about fantasies of performing fellatio and having anal intercourse with the other boys. He then proceeded to tell me that ever since he was a student in high school, he had kept a secret from the world. The secret was that he was unable to urinate or defecate in public toilets. The inhibition caused him a great deal of embarrassment and difficulty. Analysis revealed that major etiological factors contributing to his phobia of restrooms and his inhibitions in urinating and defecating in them were strong homosexual wishes to have fellatio and anal intercourse with the men in the restrooms.

Mr. A. began to examine his homosexual fantasies with less terror, and he eventually allowed himself to discuss them in his transference relationship with me. After having several dreams and fantasies in which I was "insisting" on having anal intercourse with him, he acknowledged *his own wish* to have me "insist" on having sex with him. He told me of a joke he had heard several years ago in which a man says to a young woman, "So help me, I'll rape you!" and the woman replies, "So rape me, I'll help you!" After telling me the joke, he was able to point out his identification with the woman who was being raped.

During an analytic session, after a little over a year and a half of treatment, Mr. A. described a dream in which I was raping him unmercifully. In the middle of his telling me, with obvious anxiety and embarrassment, of his wish to have me sadistically rape him, he began to giggle. When his giggling subsided, I asked him what he was thinking and feeling while he was giggling. With a note of triumph he said, "You broke the hymen, my name is————." Sounding relieved, he went on to say how much he had enjoyed teasing me, but he concluded, "Enough is enough." It should be mentioned that the patient's last name represented a punning allusion to a slang term for the female genital.

After several sessions during which Mr. A. expressed a feeling of well-being because he could tell me his name, he had a dream in which he was a teacher discussing with his students the derivation of the word "secret." Associations to the dream helped Mr. A. make his own interpretation of the dream. He pointed out the similarity between the words "secret" and "secretion" and thought that the dream was his way of making two more confessions and telling me more secrets. One confession was that he masturbated two or three times a day and enjoyed secreting a lot of sperm. He had held back telling me about his compulsive masturbation because his fantasies involved raping men and being raped by them, and this was too shameful and embarrassing to talk about. "However," Mr. A. pointed out, "when I started fantasizing raping you and being raped by you, sucking you and being sucked off by you, I thought it was time to talk about it in analysis." Mr. A. acknowledged that while his guilt, shame, and embarrassment had made him refrain from analyzing his compulsive masturbation, his holding back information from me had also made him feel powerful as he teased me. He could tease me in the way he was teased by his parents who both walked around in the nude, but never gave him very much, always holding back on him.

The other confession that Mr. A. could now make was the fact that he had been an excellent student in college but had abruptly quit as soon as the possibility of earning his degree became a reality. Analysis revealed that Mr. A. resisted telling me about his academic successes because he was afraid that I would be envious of him and then reject him. He often thought that his achievement in school activated envy and rage in his father; it was therefore something that had to be subdued or avoided altogether.

During the middle of the third year of Mr. A.'s analysis, further understanding emerged as to why he had to keep his intellectual capacities and achievements a secret. Succeeding academically or on the job was an oedipal victory that made him feel intensely guilty for being too murderous and too sexual. He pointed out that around the age of 14 when he was having many incestuous fantasies about his mother and his sister, as well as many combative and murderous fantasies about his father, his father did die suddenly. A dream during this phase of analysis revealed what Mr. A. called his biggest, deepest, and worst secret. He dreamed that his sister and mother were putting on bathrobes over their nude bodies while his father was lying on the floor, dying. Mr. A. was very apologetic as he looked at his dead father in the dream, but he could sense a note of glee in himself at the same time.

As Mr. A. got more in touch with his profound guilt about believing he had killed his father and had taken over his mother and sister, he felt more comfortable about returning to college and completing his studies. While he did complete his work, he had considerable resistance to giving up his low-paying job and bettering himself. Although Mr. A. speculated that he was afraid to become my equal, which did sound like a possibility, further analysis showed that another secret was at work. This secret, however, was less conscious. His dreams and fantasies showed that he believed that if he were successful on the job and in life, it would mean that he had completed a successful analysis. "This," pointed out Mr. A., "would give you too much satisfaction. I don't want you to feel too smug."

Mr. A.'s last year of analysis consisted primarily of examining the secret pleasure he derived from defeating me by not getting better. As he became more aware of his strong oedipal wishes to defeat me and of his deep homosexual yearning to hold onto a father figure, he could eventually terminate analysis and move on to a successful career.

In the work with Mr. A., the analysis of several countertransference reactions helped me to better understand the clinical material and to relate to the patient with more empathy. A few times during the analysis, particularly during the early phases of it, I felt irritated and teased by Mr. A. and occasionally fantasied "insisting" that he tell me his name, thus complying with his own fantasy to be forced into submission (raped). In contrast to my experience with any other patient I have ever treated, I found myself talking a great deal about the case of Mr. A. with colleagues. As I analyzed my wish to discuss him with colleagues, I got in touch with a fantasy: if I talked about the patient enough, maybe someone would know him and tell me his name! This preoccupation with Mr. A. certainly complied with his own wish to tease me and to have a father who was very concerned about and preoccupied with him.

It should also be mentioned that as I experienced frustration in not knowing Mr. A.'s secrets, I occasionally observed paranoid reactions in myself, wondering, "Who is this man, really?" A few of my colleagues also became somewhat paranoid when I discussed the case with them and wondered about the possible dangers in treating Mr. A. My paranoid reactions and those of my colleagues were again something Mr. A. unconsciously wished to happen—I should suffer and feel in danger, similar to the way he was feeling.

Finally, Mr. A.'s secretiveness, teasing, and preoccupation with sexual matters kept me very much alert with him, almost always on my toes. This posture of mine, I am sure, is one that Mr. A. craved because it gratified several wishes for him: he enjoyed teasing me because he was getting sadistic gratification from tormenting me rather than suffering himself, he had a parental figure giving him enormous attention, and he gratified himself sexually by having a father figure whom he constantly stimulated.

DISCUSSION

The dynamics of Mr. A.'s secretiveness become quite clear if we recall his dreams, fantasies, and transference reactions. Like most patients who keep secrets from their analysts, Mr. A. projected his critical superego onto me and feared my disapproval (Fine 1982, Freud 1912). However, as the clinical material demonstrates, his secretiveness encompassed many other motives, and these motives, if reviewed, provide valuable suggestions about why patients consciously withhold material from their analysts.

Mr. A. enjoyed teasing me. In effect, he was playing a popular game from childhood with me, "I've got a secret, but I won't tell." By teasing me, Mr. A. could place me in a passive, dependent position and sadistically torment me—a position he very much feared but one he unconsciously wished for himself (Brenman 1952). In teasing me, he could move from his traditional position of victim to that of victor, from passive object to powerful director. Instead of his analyst being his tormentor, I would be his slave. By teasing me, he could experience a sense of grandiosity and not feel castrated and humiliated (Stoller 1975).

One of Mr. A.'s most important motives in keeping his name a secret was an unconscious wish that I rape him. From the first session to the two hundred and seventeenth, he was extremely preoccupied with his fear that I would "insist" on his telling me his name (and "insist" on his using the couch). His fear about my insistence masked his strong unconscious wish to be raped. When he could face his wish to be raped, to be a woman who would give up her virginity, he could tell me his name.

Mr. A.'s notions about the similarity between the words "secret" and "secretion" seem quite ingenious. They parallel the notions of Bonaparte (1952) who concluded that confessing a secret was like confessing masturbation.

Keeping secrets, for Mr. A., was in many ways keeping his sexual fantasies hidden. Not only did he have to hide his wish to be a virgin woman and be raped, and not only did he have to keep his compulsive masturbation a secret, he was also holding back his incestuous wishes and his oedipal desires (Linder 1953, Reik 1957).

Mr. A.'s secret murderous wishes, coupled with his incestuous wishes (i.e., his oedipal conflict), seem to explain his wish to keep secret his academic accomplishments and his intellectual potential. Doing well academically and/or professionally was unconsciously equated in Mr. A.'s mind with destroying father and seducing mother and sister. These wishes were Mr. A.'s "biggest, deepest, and worst secret."

Finally, Mr. A. had to keep his negative therapeutic reaction (Freud 1923) a secret. He could not successfully terminate treatment until he could analyze his secret wish to defeat me and to deprive me of the gratification of curing him.

In reviewing Mr. A.'s treatment, particularly in reviewing his transference relationship with me, I found my attention drawn to the fairy tale "Rumpelstiltskin." In that story the miller falsely brags to the king that his daughter can spin straw into gold. When the king hears this, he incarcerates the girl in a room until she can spin a large quantity of gold. Helpless and panicked, the girl is saved only through the intervention of a little elf who says that he will spin the gold for her if she promises to give him her firstborn child. After the elf spins the gold, the miller's daughter reneges and does not want to give him her firstborn child. Some tense negotiations ensue, with the elf finally agreeing to forgo being the recipient of the girl's firstborn child, providing she can guess his name. When the miller's daughter correctly guesses the elf's name, the elf exclaims, "The devil has told you that!" In his anger he plunges his right foot into the earth, so much so that his whole leg goes in. A moment later, he pulls at his left leg so hard that he tears himself in two.

There are linkages between the fantasy themes in "Rumpelstiltskin" and the case of Mr. A. Pregenital, sadomasochistic themes are prominent in both.

REFERENCES

Bonaparte, M. (1952). Masturbation and death or a compulsive confession of masturbation. *Psychoanalytic Study of the Child* 7:170–172. New York: International Universities Press.

Brenman, M. (1952). On teasing and being teased: and the problem of "moral masochism." *Psychoanalytic Study of the Child* 7:264–285. New York: International Universities Press.

Complete Grimm's Fairy Tales, The (1972). New York: Random House.

Fine, R. (1982). *The Healing of the Mind: The Technique of Psychoanalytic Psychotherapy*, 2nd ed. New York: Free Press.

Freud, S. (1912). The dynamics of transference. *Standard Edition* 12:97–108.

—— (1923). The ego and the id. *Standard Edition* 19:12–68.

Lindner, R. M. (1953). *Explorations in Psychoanalysis: Essays in Honor of Theodor Reik on the Occasion of His Sixty-Fifth Birthday*. New York: Julian.

Reik, T. (1957). *The Compulsion to Confess: On the Psychoanalysis of Crime and Punishment*. New York: Farrar, Straus, & Cudahy.

Stoller, R. J. (1975). *Perversion: The Erotic Form of Hatred*. New York: Pantheon.

Discussion:
Handling Inexplicable
Resistance and
Enjoying the Challenge

Jay Offen

D r. Strean's article, "The Patient Who Would Not Tell His Name," is a great favorite of mine. Its brevity illustrates the saying "Good things come in small packages," and it contains three important contributions to the literature. First, it serves as a pocket guide to handling patient resistances. Second, it restores id psychology to its proper place of importance in the psychoanalytic armamentarium. Third, it stimulates the reader's speculation on the effect and the message names carry in terms of family expectation and family neurosis.

In this article, Dr. Strean seats us ringside for a closeup view of mainstream analysis in action when dealing with patient resistance and the powerful curative effect it can have when properly employed. From the beginning, when the patient came in teasing and tempting Dr. Strean to "insist" that his name be revealed, through the long phase of analyzing his analyst with projections, his tricks failed to divert Strean's determination to analyze him. By means of a generous revelation of how he works with patients, Strean gives us a vividly shared series of images on how to endure and handle inexplicable resistances. For instance, when he brings in a dream about Strean as a catcher on a homosexual baseball team, Dr. Strean asks mildly, "Why a catcher?" instead of "Why a homosexual team?" If that sounds too inconsequential an example, consider these theoretical principles: (1) By the way in which he frames his questions, the analyst tries to get the patient to provide more material and make the fantasies more explicit. (2) Although encouraging the patient to discuss sexual material, the analyst maintains the same attitude as when the patient discusses any other topic. To make sexual material special rather than neutral makes it too forbidden, too titillating, and therefore something to avoid.

By revealing his own enjoyment in treating this patient, Dr. Strean raises in the reader's mind the possibility that a resistance might have an enjoyable, even an admirable side to it. This man who would not tell his name has unconsciously developed an ingenious and imaginative resistance, and if one reads to the end, the resistance has in it the key to unlocking the mystery of this patient's dynamics. Since this article is as enjoyable as it is educational, one can only surmise that analyst and patient were well and evenly matched, the patient as torturer and the analyst as undercover agent who "stayed on his toes" and who found the encounters stimulating as they matched wits.

It is an oft-quoted fact that the patients enjoyed by the analyst are the ones who get better, and the patients one doesn't care for fare less well. But it is not stressed often enough how pleasurable the practice of psychoanalysis can actually be. Fine (1982) likens the admission of enjoying analytic work to confessing a feeling as forbidden as incest. Perhaps that's one reason revealing the analyst's pleasure in his work is not prominent in the literature. But the capacity to enjoy the patient is an important therapeutic point, considering that few persons who come to be analyzed were thoroughly enjoyed as children. If we find it forbidden to enjoy our patient, are we not repeating the problem of the past in the present? In any event, both this patient and analyst were actually enjoying each other (each in his own way) as the vilifications grew from "a pig in glasses" to "slavemaster" to "cocksucker." As the patient hurls his projections, Dr. Strean listens, doesn't defend himself, and deals with various resistances the patient presents, telling us as participant-observers what the patient is doing and why and what he, the analyst, is doing and why. He does not become threatened or engage in power plays. Freud, speaking of those less skillful and less knowledgeable, said that it would be quite possible that an analyst who set great store on his own knowledge could become frustrated and might, instead, punish the patient by withdrawing interest when facing too many resistances. But in this analysis of the man who would not tell his name, all's fair in love, war, and psychoanalysis. Among other things, this article is a great war story, a war story on the way to becoming a success story.

Analyzing more capably in the heat of battle is what we all strive to do. But as Shakespeare reminds us, "We are all frail." It seems only sensible to admit that an analyst can be just as uncomfortable as a patient when it appears that he's been outmaneuvered and is not in control of a situation. Yet Strean can also enjoy and make use of the uncertainty and stress involved in working with a patient so full of epithet.

This article is a lovely example of how well an analysis works when it focuses on sex and aggression, particularly in a patient in whom sex and aggression abound. One might think it abounds so obviously in this patient that no analyst could get him to talk about anything else. And yet, those of us who have had experience supervising or teaching could attest to the many ways analysts in training (and others) are capable of diverting, stultifying, or squelching id material. It takes two to let an id speak for itself.

Freud (1923) describes the analyst as afraid of doing harm by bringing the repressed sexual instincts into the patient's consciousness. He shrinks from touching the sore spot in the patient's mind for fear of increasing suffering.

Id material is too often left out of the analysis to the detriment of the patient and sometimes to the greater comfort of the analyst. Who wants to be called a rapist or cocksucker if something less volatile can be found to fill the session, especially if a theory can be produced to back up that safer thing? But in this article Dr. Strean shows how possible it is to survive the patient's hostile sexual projections while the patient begins to feel better in sessions, and then more hopeful and successful in life. Of course, this makes the good doctor feel more hopeful and successful, too. Such a strategy, we might decide, could have similar results in our own practices.

The last reason I find the article such a favorite is that stories about names have always interested me, especially what messages are carried in terms of a family's expectations and neuroses when a child is named. My interest is personal because my own name caused me great discomfort. My given and family names together were "Jay Walker," a source of amusement to my classmates in school. I never liked to tell anyone my name, particularly when somebody may have joked about it. Dr. Strean's patient refused to tell his name, in part because it referred to something sexual and in part because it was open to ridicule. It was not until the patient had resolved his resistances to his forbidden aggressive and sexual wishes that he could consider divulging his name to his analyst. By helping the patient resolve his struggles as shown in the transference, Strean could then be privileged to know the patient's name.

Perhaps what I most enjoy about this article is that it is very human. We do not get to see or hear about the analyst's doubts, frustrations, and furies with this patient, but we can assume them as being a part of any intense analysis. What we do get to see and to carry away with us is the ongoing dedication to the patient, no matter what, and the strong sense that Dr. Strean found pleasure in the work where another analyst might find only pain. That's a good lesson.

As I was writing this paper, a patient I have been seeing for several months told me she had decided to change her first name. Then she folded her arms and said, "But I'm not going to tell you what new name I've chosen. I don't want you to know." I felt like looking over my shoulder to see if Dr. Strean and his patient were somewhere just behind me, taking in the scene. There are such elusive and unknowable elements in the countertransference that it couldn't be mere coincidence to suddenly be facing a patient who would not tell me her name. Indeed, Freud has taught us that coincidence cannot exist in psychoanalysis. What had I revealed or stimulated in her to help cause this situation? I can only wonder. Several sessions later, after exploring together why she might like keeping a secret from me, she said, "Okay, I'll tell you. I want to be called Jamie. It's the name of my father's favorite brother, who died young. Sometimes my Dad would call me that." The name Jamie also contains my name. "Jay . . . me" Perhaps "Jay and me . . ." or "Jay/me . . . me/Jay . . ." This name could contain libidinal wishes of which the patient is not yet aware. As our work together unfolds, I will keep Dr. Strean's article in mind and remember to enjoy the challenge.

REFERENCES

Fine, R. (1982). *The Healing of the Mind*, 2nd ed. New York: Free Press.

Freud, S. (1923). The ego and the id. *Standard Edition* 19:3–66.

Discussion:
Secrets as a Special
Form of Resistance

Stephen Weiss

Individuals typically enter psychotherapy because they are feeling unhappy or unfulfilled and are seeking greater satisfaction in their lives. A basic premise of psychoanalysis or psychoanalytically oriented psychotherapy is that maladaptive functioning is the result of underlying psychic conflicts. Change can occur only when those conflicts are recognized and resolved. Therefore, the patient is asked to free associate, that is, to speak openly and honestly about his thoughts, feelings, dreams, and behavior, no matter how odd they may seem, so that the therapist can understand the problems and be of help. Almost from the beginning, however, the patient tries to thwart the therapeutic process in both subtle and obvious ways. Therapists are confronted with the paradox that, despite expressing a desire to improve their existence, patients resist change in order to protect themselves from the anxieties aroused by facing unpleasant truths in therapy. As well, patients distort the relationship with the therapist in the present by acting toward the therapist in a manner similar to the way they behaved with significant persons from their past. This happens as patients experience fantasies, wishes, and impulses toward the therapist that are a repetition and displacement of reactions to important persons in their early childhood. To make the work more complex, therapists have their own reactions to patients' styles of resisting and relating to them. To the extent that therapists are unaware of patients' effects on them, their decisions about how best to work therapeutically are compromised. The therapist's task is to analyze patients' transference and resistance phenomena, in an atmosphere of self-awareness and reflection, so that the patient can gain insight into the psychic conflicts and work them through.

In this context, Dr. Herb Strean's paper, "The Patient Who Would Not Tell His Name," is a vivid study of Mr. A., a 34-year-old man in psychoanalysis who consciously kept secrets as a means of avoiding or withholding material, a "special form of resistance, the handling of which requires particular technical considerations" (Greenson 1967, p. 68). While patients may have different motivations for keeping secrets, in this case Mr. A. wanted to torture his analyst sadistically and, through the transference neurosis, enacted murderous, incestuous wishes growing from an intense oedipal conflict. Several major themes arise from the case: the value of analyzing, and not colluding with, the patient's wish to keep secrets; the role of superego projections and role reversal in secretive behavior; the sexual, oedipal conflicts that made keeping the secret so necessary; and the importance of examining countertransference issues to promote therapeutic understanding. These themes will be discussed briefly.

While all patients have memories buried in their unconscious that are kept secret from their conscious awareness, patients who purposefully withhold information of any kind jeopardize the success of their treatment. Freud (1913) described his experience attempting to analyze a ranking government official who refused to discuss certain state issues in the analysis. When Freud permitted the secrets, the analysis failed. He compared the analyst's allowing secrets to a situation where the police were not exercising their power in one part of a village. Soon that area would become a refuge where all the rascals would assemble and escape detection. Freud asserted that all secrets, no matter what their content, needed to be analyzed because any secret could become a screen that protected all the patient's forbidden thoughts, memories, and impulses.

Greenson (1967) affirms that secrets need to be considered as resistance that must be analyzed but are "to be respected and not crushed, coerced, or begged out of the patient" (p. 68). He points out that while refusing to tell the secret is a conscious act, the true reasons for maintaining the secrecy are unconscious and the analyst's goal is to make the patient aware of the underlying motives. He states:

> In general, secrets are related to secretions. They always have some anal or urethral connotation, and are considered shameful and loathsome, or its opposite, that is very valuable and to be hoarded and protected. Secrets are also connected to the parents' secret sexual activities, which now the patient repeats via identification and which the patient does in revenge in the transference situation. In addition to all of this, secrecy and confession are always involved with problems of exhibitionism, scoptophilia, and teasing. The secret is inevitably involved in the transference situation as a special form of resistance. [p. 133]

Jacobs (1980) suggests that because "the word 'secret' is derived from the same root as 'secretions' and because of the secretive nature of the bodily processes . . . secrets are closely linked in the mind with issues of control and power" (p. 34). Withholding a secret is linked to control of the body, particularly sphincter control, and is experienced as an act of aggression.

Fine (1982) pointed out that all patients have secrets, and starting with Freud's patients until the present, as patient is exempt from them.

Anna Freud (1966) describes the case of a young woman patient who angrily accused her therapist of being secretive. She wanted the therapist to reveal more about her personal life and was hurt when the therapist was silent. The demands would cease for a short time, only to resume again. However, the patient was keeping secrets of her own and, by doing so, knew that she was breaking the fundamental rule of analysis. Consequently, she expected the analyst to reprimand her. Noting that the patient's periods of aggressiveness toward her therapist correlated with her phases of secretiveness, Anna Freud states that the patient "introjected the fantasied rebuke and, adopting the active role, applied the accusation to the analyst . . . She criticized the analyst for the very fault of which she herself was guilty. Her own secretive behavior was perceived as reprehensible conduct on the analyst's part" (p. 117). Anna Freud presents this case to exemplify the defensive reaction known as *identification with the aggressor*, a phase of superego development that includes (1) the child introjecting the characteristics of the person that are felt as threatening, (2) the child identifying with that person and imitating his threatening behavior, and (3) projecting that threatening behavior externally, thus coping with anxiety by transforming herself from being passively threatened to actively threatening others.

The dynamics described above were at work in the psychoanalysis of Mr. A. As treatment began, the patient was afraid of his angry and destructive feelings toward the father whom he experienced as demanding and disapproving. He "depressed" those feelings and appeared deferential and compliant in the initial consultation. However, as he did with all authority figures, Mr. A. immediately turned Dr. Strean into the dominant and controlling father and proceeded to make the transference into a power struggle. Mr. A. attempted to psychologically castrate Dr. Strean by refusing to give his name, lie on the couch, or pay the fee by check. By "standing up" to what he thought the analyst would "insist" upon, the patient was defending against his homosexual fears. Dr. Strean accepted the patient's provocative attempts to reduce his power without countertransference needs to assert his authority and demand that the patient follow the analytic "rules." Instead, the analyst restrained his emotional reactions and was able to listen neutrally without feeling "neutered." When Dr. Strean was able to recognize, clarify, and interpret that the patient was experiencing the analyst and his employers in the way he remembered his father, the initial resistances diminished.

Paranoid projections were present throughout the analysis. Mr. A. formed a transference in which he turned Dr. Strean into the aggressor and consistently attributed his own sexual and aggressive feelings to the analyst. According to Mr. A.'s transference projections, it was the analyst who wanted to tease and be raped, who had strong homosexual yearnings, and who envied Mr. A.'s success. The analyst did not react with counteraggression nor did he try to avoid the patient's emotions by placating or trying to soothe him. A strong working alliance emerged that gradually permitted the patient to discharge his warded-off feelings and impulses in a safe and secure environment without fear of retribution. As Dr. Strean confronted the transference displacements from the patient's father to himself, accepted and clarified the paranoid distortions, and interpreted the patient's transference resistances, the therapy progressed. Mr. A. gradually felt relief and eventually yielded his name.

Strengthening of the therapeutic alliance brought dreams, jokes, childhood history, and confessions about his intense oedipal rivalry and homosexual impulses toward the analyst/ father. Revelations about bigger and deeper secrets emerged as the analysis grew in length and depth. The patient was able to disclose masturbatory and rape fantasies, sexual thoughts about his mother and sister, and death wishes toward the father that came true. The termination phase brought new competitive struggles with the analyst in which progressing in treatment meant losing to the analyst and loss of him. As Dr. Strean interpreted and worked through the patient's need to defeat the analyst, while, at the same time, having intense wishes for a good father figure, the analysis came to an end.

Calef and Weinshel (1981) discuss the efforts of individuals to influence others by causing the latter to doubt their judgment. In a number of clinical examples, persons who were the recipients of such behavior tended to incorporate what others projected onto them. Similar events may happen in the analytic setting. Analysts inevitably become the targets for patients' unacceptable feelings and conflicts. "Since those feelings and conflicts are often universal, analysts may not find it easy to separate what the patients wrongly ascribe to them from what truly belongs to them" (Calef and Weinshel 1981, p. 54).

Pick (1985) suggests that patients attempt to elicit an "enacting response" in the analytic situation, that is, to induce the analyst to meet their expressed needs, rather than examine those needs more deeply. On their side, analysts may have the impulse to respond in just that way through interpretations and nonanalytic behaviors. Thus, a patient's need for mothering coincides with a part of the analyst that needs to be a mother, while, at another point, the patient's wish to avoid recognizing fears of death matches the analyst's own deep-rooted anxieties. Pick's perspective suggests that the patient is as likely to influence the therapist as the opposite. In such cases, therapeutic impasse may result if analysts cannot work through their countertransference reactions.

All analysts have transference reactions to their patients because therapy is an interaction between two individuals. We refer to the therapist's responses to the patient as *counter-transference* only to distinguish between the two participants in the analytic dyad. Patients with powerful infantile needs may elicit more intense reactions from the therapist; however, the therapist must experience such countertransference reactions in order to understand the transference dynamics and be able to interpret them to the patient (McLaughlin 1981). In Mr. A.'s case, the fear that he would be forced into giving his name arose from his homosexual wishes to be forced into submission. As the patient externalized these paranoid fantasies in the transference, he teased and irritated the analyst to the point where Dr. Strean almost demanded that the name be given. Thus, Mr. A. tried to induce the analyst to satisfy his unconscious wishes to be raped. In identifying with the analyst's position, I marveled at the equanimity that Dr. Strean showed during the sessions in the face of the patient's sadism and wondered that he did not reveal his countertransference responses to the patient under duress.

Mr. A.'s needs to have a concerned father and to be the center of attention were also enacted in the therapy as Dr. Strean became preoccupied by thoughts about the patient and involved other therapists in his countertransference struggles. Dr. Strean apparently hoped that discussing Mr. A. with colleagues might elicit recognition from another therapist who would supply the patient's name. I question whether the patient's wishes for attention and fathering were being induced as part of the countertransference as the analyst found himself seeking the assistance of other authorities for his own needs. While Dr. Strean does not indicate whether he disclosed his countertransference feelings as part of the treatment process, and whether it was helpful, his awareness and management of both transference and countertransference led to a successful outcome of the analysis. Clearly, Mr. A. was a very stimulating patient.

Dr. Strean's cogent study illustrates the value of understanding theory in the context of practice. It also highlights the importance of analysts examining their countertransference responses to better understand the clinical material and to relate to the patient with more empathy. As Reed (1996) states, "Although theory is an invaluable organizer of a clinician's perceptions, it doesn't tell one what to do in the clinical moment . . . for that one must rely on one's own capacity for self-understanding as that capacity has been sharpened by experience, including, most importantly, one's own analyses" (p. xvi).

Bernfeld (1941), in his classic "The Facts of Observation in Psychoanalysis," observed that the patient's divulging of a secret tended to follow a comment of the analyst that conveyed acceptance and thereby diminished in the patient internal shame or distrust. The psychotherapy research of Sampson and Weiss (1986) has independently confirmed and expanded on Bernfeld's perception. In addition, it tends to explain how Dr. Strean's accepting attitidue helped Mr. A. divulge his secrets.

REFERENCES

Bernfeld, S. (1941). The facts of observation in psychoànalysis. *International Review of Psycho-Analysis* 12:342–351.

Calef, V., and Weinshel, E. (1981). Some clinical consequences of introjection: gaslighting. *Psychoanalytic Quarterly* 50: 44–65.

Fine, R. (1982). *The Healing of the Mind*, 2nd ed. New York: Free Press.

Freud, A. (1966). *The Ego and the Mechanisms of Defence*. New York: International Universities Press.

Freud, S. (1913). On beginning the treatment. *Standard Edition* 12:121–144.

Greenson, R. (1967). *The Technique and Practice of Psychotherapy*. New York: International Universities Press.

Jacobs, T. (1980). Secrets, alliances, and family fictions: some psychoanalytic observations. *Journal of the American Psychoanalytic Association* 28: 21–42.

McLaughlin, J. (1981). Transference, psychic reality, and

countertransference. *Psychoanalytic Quarterly* 50:639–654.

Pick, I. (1985). Working through in the countertransference. *International Journal of Psycho-Analysis* 66:157–166.

Reed, G. (1996). *Clinical Understanding*. Northvale, NJ: Jason Aronson.

Sampson, H., and Weiss, J. (1986). *The Psychoanalytic Process: Theory, Clinical Observation, and Empirical Research*. New York: Guilford.

Sandler, J. (1976). Countertransference and role responsiveness. *International Review of Psychoanalysis* 7:43–47.

Epilogue

As I tried to identify with you, the reader of this text, I asked myself repeatedly, "What is the best way to conclude this book?" Inasmuch as I could not come up with any definitive answer, I tried to understand what my hesitancy was all about. Eventually, it dawned on me that my indecision was a reflection of my realization that many of the controversies on countertransference are not settled—at least not for me! Notions like self-disclosure of the countertransference continue to be debated. Can countertransference reactions be reliably used to tell us about the patient's internal dynamics? How much gratification should the therapist receive in the treatment situation? How much pain does he have to endure? Are we all wounded healers? These and other questions are far from fully resolved.

But after carefully reading and rereading the twelve discussants' remarks, and after reviewing my own contribution to this volume, I believe we can say several things about countertransference with some certainty. Although my twelve colleagues and I are probably not modal representatives of the mental health professions, it may be worthwhile to consider just what the thirteen therapists in this book have in common. Where are we in agreement?

First and foremost, we can concur that we have come a long way since Freud averred that countertransference interfered with the therapy and should be vanquished as soon as possible. Countertransference is here to stay! It is a universal phenomenon that never leaves any therapist and plays an active part in his or her theoretical predilections, treatment decisions, and therapeutic interventions. A corollary of this finding is that conducting psychotherapy, while based on scientific principles, is an art that always involves the therapist's subjectivity—her fantasies, memories, defenses, and superego injunctions. The days of the wise and "together" therapist working with the troubled, "not together" patient are over. Both practitioner and patient are "more human than otherwise" and are equal partners in a shared enterprise.

Although therapist and patient have different roles, both are consciously and unconsciously striving to induce the other to enact behaviors that will gratify and support the inducer. When these role sets are congruent and complementary, the treatment is usually in a state of equilibrium—but the patient may not grow much. For example, if the patient wants to become the admired child of the therapist, and the latter elects to admire, a love-and-be-loved relationship might ensue but with little therapeutic movement. However, if the therapist responds to the patient's demands for admiration with interpretations, the patient may feel frustrated, respond with anger, challenge the practitioner, and may threaten him or her with termination of the treatment. These episodes or treatment crises constitute the heart of most good therapies and activate many transference and countertransference reactions.

Because countertransference struggles can only be viewed with clarity after the fact, it does take time before we can be sure just what we are feeling toward our patients and how we are constructively or destructively influencing them. Once we do recognize how our patients are affecting us and we them, what countertransference reactions can we share with them? Minimally, we can agree that when resistances are intractable and interpretations yield negative therapeutic reactions, the therapist's hurt, frustration, disappointment, and anger often can be profitably shared with the patient, and solid therapeutic movement usually ensues. Very often cases remain intractable because the therapist is unwilling to share some of his subjective reactions that have led to mutual misunderstanding.

When countertransference responses are shared with the patient, the test of their validity is how the patient reacts to the disclosure. If the therapeutic alliance is strengthened and therapeutic movement ensues, the disclosure was probably on the money. The test of any intervention's therapeutic utility can only be revealed by a careful observation of the patient's transference reactions, dreams, fantasies, and overall behavior in the therapy situation.

As the therapist demonstrates that he is capable of error, can tolerate a wide range of emotions in himself, and demonstrates these very human qualities with the patient, the patient feels safer to become a feeling, reacting, object-related person. The therapist's abstaining, trying to be neutral and anonymous, often interferes with the patient's growth as she feels obligated to submit to an authoritarian, punitive superego.

As countertransference has become a dynamic reality in the treatment situation, it is now utilized more and more in supervision and in the classroom. Just as the therapist can learn from the patient, so too, the supervisor can learn from the supervisee. There is a declining authoritarianism in psychotherapy, supervision, and education for mental health professionals. This attitude individualizes the patient more and seems to be leading to more promising therapeutic results.

All of the participants in this study recognize that there is a child very much alive in all patients and all therapists. This child progresses and regresses all of the time, and treatment, supervision, and education always have their ups and downs. When therapists, patients, students and teachers, supervisors and supervisees accept with more and more equanimity the child in themselves and the child in those with whom they frequently interact, life will yield more pleasure and fulfillment for all of us.

I believe that most of the participants in this study would agree with what Schafer (2000) has postulated—namely, that each person has a hand in creating that which he seems only to encounter; that persons, situations, and events are neither pure reality nor pure subjectivity or fantasy; that psychoanalysis and psychotherapy create and discover in one and the same act. Thus, both therapist and patient are continuously constructing their individually experienced situations. However, this does not imply, as one or two of my colleagues suggest, that there can only be encounters of two subjective realities in what is implicitly a completely solipsistic universe. As a psychoanalyst, Schafer (2000) states it thus:

> This claim contains a paradox. For it is the analyst who keeps the record and the frame of the analytic work; it is the analyst who steadily tries to affirm and integrate and safeguard the treatment and the analysand. Furthermore, it is the analyst who gives the final account of the analysis and sustains what we have agreed to call the reality of psychoanalysis. [p. 17]

REFERENCE

Schafer, R. (2000). *Tradition and Change in Psychoanalysis*. Madison, CT: International Universities Press.

Credits

Index

About the Editor

Herbert S. Strean, D. S. W., was Distinguished Professor Emeritus, Rutgers University School of Social Work, and Director Emeritus of the New York Center for Psychoanalytic Training. Author of thirty-five books and over one hundred professional articles, his most recent books include *The Extramarital Affair* (2000), *Don't Lose Your Patients: Responding to Clients Who Want to Quit Treatment* (1998), *When Nothing Else Works: Innovative Interventions with Intractable Individuals* (1998), *Mending the Broken Heart* (1996), *Psychotherapy with the Unattached* (1995), *Psychotherapy with the Orthodox Jew* (1994), and *Jokes: Their Purpose and Meaning* (1993). Dr. Strean served on the editorial boards of *Psychoanalytic Review*, *Clinical Social Work*, *Current Issues in Psychoanalytic Practice*, and *Psychoanalytic Social Work*.

The recipient of many honors and awards, Dr. Strean trained over 4,000 therapists in his more than forty-five years of professional practice. He lectured extensively on psychotherapeutic and mental health issues in the United States and Canada. Dr. Strean maintained a private practice in psychotherapy and supervision in New York City.